MUM, PLEASE HELP ME!

KAREN PERKS

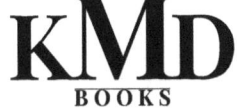

Copyright © KMD Books
First published in Australia in 2024
by KMD Books
Waikiki, WA 6169

Copyright © 2025 Karen Perks

All rights reserved. No part of this book may be used or reproduced by any means, graphic, electronic, or mechanical, including photocopying, recording, taping or by any information storage retrieval system without the written permission of the copyright owner except in the case of brief quotations embodied in critical articles and reviews.

Because of the dynamic nature of the Internet, any web addresses or links contained in this book may have changed since publication and may no longer be vaild. The views expressed in this work are solely those of the author and do not necessarily reflect the views of the publisher and the publisher hereby disclaims any responsibility for them.

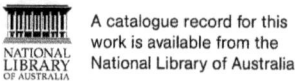

A catalogue record for this work is available from the National Library of Australia

National Library of Australia Catalogue-in-Publication data:
Mum, Please Help Me / Karen Perks

DEDICATION

To my courageous children, whose steadfast spirit has guided us through the darkest times, this book serves as a tribute to your resilience, strength, and unending love, which unites our family amid unimaginable challenges.

I also dedicate this to all families who have faced the pain and frustration of medical misdiagnosis, reminding them that their voices matter and that their fight for accurate care is not in vain.

May this story inspire hope, empower advocacy, and ultimately contribute to a future in which every patient receives the timely and appropriate treatment they deserve. May our story also convey that adversity can foster strength, resilience, and unity.

This is for those who feel unheard, unseen, and overlooked. Remember that your experiences and feelings are valid, and your struggles deserve acknowledgment.

We stand by you, will fight for you, and shall continue to fight for every family facing a similar struggle.

"It's given me time to think about life, and what the true value of love and joy is, and that it is, rarely, rarely, rarely tied to anything financial."
Dan Levy

DISCLAIMER

"This book draws on our personal experiences navigating the healthcare system. Although we faced significant challenges, we also recognise the dedication of many medical professionals who work tirelessly under difficult conditions. Our aim is not to criticise individuals, but to highlight systemic issues that affect patient care, hoping to improve future outcomes for others."

CONTENTS

Preface 1
Introduction 3

PART ONE
Chapter 1: The beginning 7
Chapter 2: The growing frequency of seizures 13
Chapter 3: Twenty-one visits and counting 20
Chapter 4: Thirty different doctors 28
Chapter 5: The timeline 36
Chapter 6: What will we do? 41

PART TWO
Chapter 7: Through Mikayla's Eyes 49
Chapter 8: Through Alana's Eyes 58
Chapter 9: Through Karen's eyes 64
Chapter 10: Family, friends, and neighbours 69

PART THREE
Chapter 11: Balancing mental health with managing health risks 77
Chapter 12: Parental intuition and research 88

Chapter 13: AI and medical diagnosis – is this the future? 94
Chapter 14: How we used AI in Mikayla's diagnosis process 101
Chapter 15: Compelling data ignored 106
Chapter 16: Difficult conversations with doctors.. 111

PART FOUR
Chapter 17: The wild and wonderful comments.. 119
Chapter 18: Patient advocacy... 122
Chapter 19: Complaints and formal grievances.. 126
Chapter 20: Exploring options for accountability......................................131
Chapter 21: Bullying and gaslighting 134
Chapter 22: Strategies for self-preservation 137

PART FIVE
Chapter 23: An accurate diagnosis finally revealed.................................... 143
Chapter 24: Mikayla and the family today... 153
Chapter 25: Resilience through courage 158
Chapter 26: Being grateful 165
Chapter 27: Thank you to you 169

PART SIX
Chapter 28: The importance of having your patient records 177
Chapter 29: Eight specialties and counting... 181
Chapter 30: But why did this happen? 184
Chapter 31: The financial cost is to everybody 186

PART SEVEN
Chapter 32: Evolution of the medical profession 193
Chapter 33: Why do organisations like healthcare fail us? 204
Chapter 34: How can we use technology to help the medical profession? ..211

Chapter 35: Hospital structures and Mikayla's medical misdiagnosis 214
Chapter 36: What needs to change first to address medical misdiagnosis . 220

PART EIGHT
Chapter 37: Lessons learnt from the journey 233
Chapter 38: Inspiring others to speak up 238
Chapter 39: Where to from here? 241
Chapter 40: The personal thank you... 244

Glossary 246
Author Biography 248

PREFACE

Brené Brown, one of my favourite authors, once said: "One day, you'll share your story of how you overcame what you went through, and it will be someone else's survival guide." This idea inspired our family to write this book and strive to transform a system burdened by structural flaws.

When my daughter had her first seizure, we entered a realm of medicine that presented a bewildering array of specialists and a misdiagnosis overlooked by those in authority. I frequently questioned: if I feel lost and unheard, how do those struggling to navigate or advocate for themselves succeed?

This is the book you will need when you least expect it.

During the 18 months, the medical system continually challenged Mikayla and our family. Doctors, nurses, and other healthcare professionals were caught in a culture of blame, hierarchy, mistrust, and unrealistic expectations of perfection.

We made twenty-one trips to the accident and emergency department, consulted with thirty different doctors, whilst Mikayla endured two hundred seizures. Our family faced a system that appeared designed to let us down.

Every dismissal and every trivialised concern chipped away at our hope, putting us under immense emotional and financial burdens. Through difficult lessons, we frequently learned the importance of relentless advocacy and careful documentation while facing the subtle but harmful impacts of medical gaslighting.

How has a system deteriorated to the point where it cannot operate without restrictions? This model is beset by dysfunction, ineffective communication, and an inability to function correctly and adapt.

This book shares our journey while serving as a guide for families navigating the challenging landscape of undiagnosed and misdiagnosed medical issues. Within these pages, you will learn about our experiences and uncover valuable insights into complex systems, escalation strategies, and resources designed to assist you in finding your voice to advocate effectively for your loved ones.

We aspire for this book to inspire hope and remind you that you are not alone, and that the truth can shine through with determination. Our intention in writing this book is to guide you through the intricacies of the healthcare system and empower you to advocate effectively for the best care for your loved ones. By recounting our experiences, we hope to spare other families from enduring the same pain and challenges we faced. We also aim to inspire hope through advocacy, change, and future advancements in medical diagnosis.

INTRODUCTION

"Mum, please help me!" is more than just a book title – it was a frequent plea. How many times did she say these words? How many times did her eyes ask the question? It broke my heart each time.

I can feel the weight of our responsibility in shaping our narrative. This story must be shared with others who have had similar experiences worldwide, a narrative wherein a safeguarded system remains unchanged.

For us, it represents a time of 21 visits to the emergency department, 30 doctors, 200 seizures, a loss of confidence in the medical system, and a continual disregard for our increasing concerns and mounting evidence that the diagnosis was incorrect.

This book explores our journey through a healthcare system that at times appeared indifferent to Mikayla's suffering. It captures not only the medical challenges we faced but also the emotional toll, financial strain, and overwhelming sense of helplessness that frequently accompany medical misdiagnosis.

We aim to highlight the systemic flaws that can lead to such failures through detailed accounts of emergency room visits, consultations with various specialists, and the ongoing struggle for an accurate diagnosis.

Our narrative will provide valuable insights into the challenges confronted by the system, communication strategies, escalation techniques, methods for protecting mental health, and resources available for families encountering similar difficulties.

We aim to provide readers with the essential tools to navigate the complexities of the healthcare system and advocate for their rights and the well-being of their loved ones.

This story illustrates resilience, a family's steadfast love, and the urgent need for improved patient care in complex health conditions. It serves as a testament to the importance of perseverance, even when faced with significant challenges, and advocates for a more responsive and accountable healthcare system. Every patient deserves to be heard, understood, and treated with dignity and compassion.

This book represents our contribution to this vital cause. May it catalyse discussion and a movement, ensuring that no family must endure the suffering we experienced.

"Fear that turned into courage – darkness that turned to light.
Lives that have taken a turn – stronger and more courageous than ever."
Karen Perks

PART ONE

PART ONE

CHAPTER 1

THE BEGINNING

The day ended like any other – 11 pm on a Friday, and Mikayla had left for work; the house was quiet, and the week was over. Peace and tranquillity enveloped the space, asleep and dreaming. I could hear someone's phone ringing. Could you answer it, please? Then, a sudden realisation – it was my phone.

It was now 12:10 a.m. I sat up quickly, thinking that no one would call at this time of night. Looking at my phone, I realised it was Mikayla's number. I thought there had better be a good reason for her to call. She knew I would be asleep, but she also knew I would answer.

It wasn't Mikayla, though. The voice sounded off. I was waking up quickly, attempting to understand why Mikayla's store manager had called me on her phone. "What's wrong?" I asked. That was the only reason her workplace would contact me in the middle of the night. Something must be serious.

"Mikayla has collapsed and is having a seizure."

Panic, raw and visceral, seized me. What was happening, I wondered? This had never happened before. "Where is she?" I asked. The restaurant floor was the reply: "Have you called an ambulance?" "Yes," came the response. I'm on my way," I said.

I leapt out of bed, threw on my clothes, and dashed to my car. The seven-kilometre journey seemed to last an eternity. My heart pounded—a frantic drumbeat of fear.

The ambulance paramedics bombarded me with questions, yet I had more questions than answers. She slowly regained consciousness and was taken to the emergency department.

I called my eldest daughter, my voice choking with fear. I could scarcely articulate the event that had unfolded before my eyes. "Be strong," my mind kept repeating.

When I arrived at the ED, she had been triaged and sent to the waiting room. Why are we in the waiting room? Hours later, she is called. We go back behind "the wall." I call it the wall because that's where the activity occurs—another 12 hours before a doctor attends and orders a range of tests. The initial diagnosis is straightforward, almost too straightforward: fainting, and we are sent home. "Go to your GP," we are told, with discharge papers in hand. "It will likely pass." The relief was immense, a wave washing away my fear. It is common for young women to seize. We could go home. We clung to that hope, that simple explanation, like a lifeline amidst the raging turmoil of the sea.

Perusing the discharge papers provided no clarity regarding what had transpired. Essential details appeared absent, yet what can one do with such scant information following an eventful night? The relief turned out to be fleetingly short-lived.

Mikayla visited the GP and rested, but two days later, while at home, she experienced another seizure. An ambulance was called, resulting in the same questions and outcome. Off to the hospital, although it was a different local one.

After triage, she is taken to the waiting room. She collapses while seated in the waiting room chair and begins to seize again. What is happening? Where is the assistance? We gently lower her to the ground, cradling her head to prevent it from hitting the floor. 'I wouldn't recommend placing her on the floor,' the nursing staff says from behind the triage desk—it's dirty. 'How about getting some help?' is my quick retort.

Behind the ED wall, we venture. Apathy, dismissiveness, and a condescending attitude led to a disputed diagnosis of "syncope" – a complex term for fainting. Her fainting episodes were unlike any I had previously witnessed. With erratic body movements, I felt that something was amiss.

But I did say this happened two days ago. Weren't you paying attention?

We have now experienced two seizure events. I wonder if this indicates a pattern. The medical personnel are dismissive of this notion. Please consult your GP and refrain from driving for four weeks.

Feeling shocked, disheartened, and let down by the system, I submitted my first complaint to the Health Care Complaints Commission (HCCC). It was of no assistance.

Four days later, at the end of June, Mikayla began seizing at home once again while lying in bed and resting. What is happening? The realisation that this is now a pattern frightens me and sends chills down my spine. My stomach is churning.

New symptoms include tachycardia and multiple five-minute seizures. Things are changing. This time, triaging to the waiting room is no longer necessary. Instead, we ramp into the ED behind the wall. Ramping occurs when there are too many patients for the number of beds. The ambulance takes the patient to the ED, but it's a different waiting area.

I hate ramping. You cannot see the patient or your family, leaving you to sit in the waiting room for hours, wondering, worrying, and without any information.

The third time in ten days raised sufficient concerns for doctors to investigate. They acknowledged this was enough to warrant her admission to cardiology. My naivety regarding the health system caught up, and I was completely oblivious. You feel like you're on a hamster wheel, with the hospital system dictating the pace. Family involvement is limited, and the doctors provide no insights into their reasoning behind the "why" – nothing.

They stand at the end of the bed, hiding behind the patient chart clutched tightly against their chest – your loved one's life – and offer a solution. Their diagnosis. But how did you reach that diagnosis? You don't need to know. Just see how clever we are!

We spent ten days in hospital. I set up my remote office in Mikayla's room and commandeered a tray table so I could work and be there for her, often just sitting. I waited for the doctors to arrive, listening to them and attempting to read between their mumbles; typically, what they weren't saying provided the most significant clues.

Although she was admitted to cardiology, she suffered a seizure in the ward. This triggered an internal emergency, prompting the rapid response team to arrive. Seizure medications were administered, but they proved ineffective. This should have been documented as a significant clue, yet for the next nine months, doctors continued to prescribe futile drugs. Hindsight is invaluable only when one questions the results of the outcome.

Four doctors made significant statements during Mikayla's journey that should have altered the trajectory. The first occasion involved requesting a consultation with a neurology specialist in the cardiology ward. In Mikayla's room, the doctor remarked that it was unlikely to be a neurological cause. However, let's do some tests to confirm. Okay, we understand you need to eliminate anything sinister. Thank you; that made complete sense.

Mikayla was sent to neurology for further testing to exclude epilepsy. All neurological assessments yielded negative results, including those for epilepsy. Consequently, we understood she would be moved back if the issue wasn't neurological. This is when the "it's not my organ" game started. Since it isn't a cardiological issue, we can't transfer her there. This was my first time caught between specialties—the "too-hard" basket, as we call it. That concluded the discussion.

This marks the moment the system starts to fail Mikayla. It influences the following 17 ED visits and distorts every future doctor's evaluation. The doctors incorrectly diagnosed her, rushing to a diagnosis that should not have been prioritised. Such a quick conclusion was unwarranted.

On the afternoon of the ninth day, I sat quietly with my laptop when a junior doctor entered. "We have a diagnosis," he announced. He handed me some brochures and assuredly mentioned functional neurological disorder, or FND, previously known as pseudo seizures. I had difficulty absorbing the information quickly—these seizures stem from underlying psychological issues. "Are you kidding?" I questioned, though it felt more like a declaration. Not this child—there's no trauma. No one asked if any past trauma might be a trigger.

Oh, and she won't be driving for 12 months. I can see the tears welling in Mikayla's eyes. She is coming to terms with her life as she knew it, which is now gone.

He turns to leave. "Hang on," I say. "Where are you going? How can you leave that with us and walk away?"

I frantically Googled the diagnosis while trying to absorb the contents of his brochure. The brochure was well-written, yet its clarity only deepened my confusion. It clearly outlined that there are multiple types of seizures, and even with a glance, I made an unsettling realisation – they hadn't ruled out seizures caused by underlying physical conditions.

There are two categories of non-epileptic seizures: the FND category and the physiological category. Have you not considered any physical causes? How can you immediately conclude that a psychological cause is the diagnosis?

"I recommend you arrange for her psychological therapy," he said. "Her age group is more susceptible to FND seizures." "Who stated that?" I asked. This is when everything turned very serious and went from bad to worse.

CHAPTER 2

THE GROWING FREQUENCY OF SEIZURES

Days turned into weeks, then months, and the seizures continued. Their occurrence became more frequent and severe. Each time she was taken to the hospital, we braced ourselves for the same frantic atmosphere of the emergency room. The reaction was always the same: she had previously been diagnosed with functional neurological disorder (FND), and they advised us to accept this diagnosis and try some mindfulness practices.

Yet, the seizures still happen even when she engages in mindfulness activities such as watching the sunset or walking the dog. How could a sunset over a beautiful lake trigger a seizure? How can this possibly make sense? The seizures did not stop. They did not lessen. They escalated.

What began as one or two seizures had, by the fourth month, escalated into clusters of over 14 seizures, each lasting 10 to 15 minutes, with her most prolonged period of unconsciousness extending to 22 hours.

The ER felt like our second home. The doctors' and nurses' faces merged into a blur of care, yet they ultimately proved unhelpful. We found ourselves in a maze of mixed opinions and ignored worries. My insistence that it wasn't FND seemed to fall on deaf ears.

My once-organised life had been reduced to a chaotic scramble of emergency departments, sleepless nights, and increasing despair. The financial strain began to mount. Each hospital visit, and time away from work chipped away at my business, costing hundreds of thousands of dollars in lost revenue. This forced me to make difficult choices, sacrificing things that were once taken for granted, making positions redundant, and scaling down the business purposefully.

The emotional burden was even heavier. Sleep turned into a rare luxury. A trip to the ED could be extended to 24 hours if Mikayla wasn't discharged. Juggling an entire workday with 24 to 36 hours in emergency care was exhausting. This relentless fatigue took a toll, leaving us physically and emotionally drained. Worry, guilt, and a deep sense of helplessness overwhelmed us.

Without realising it, I had begun to avoid making appointments after 3 pm on Mondays and Wednesdays. Jokingly, I would tell my clients and staff that Mikayla would likely be having a seizure, and I would be at the hospital.

Yet, a common theme emerged. One Sunday, after Mikayla's discharge, we found it hard to return home. Let's visit your aunty and uncle to process everything. While enjoying a cup of tea, I casually mentioned that I blank out my diary on specific days to prepare for the phone call. Certain activities could trigger seizures or happen after a set number of days. Their advice was to maintain a comprehensive record of everything. And a massive thank you for that afternoon tea.

We started documenting Mikayla's life, recording her activities and the dates and times of these events. She had already reduced her working hours and responsibilities, taking on lighter duties and was not permitted to enter any high-risk areas of the restaurant. I set up an Excel spreadsheet to log her life, noting the day, time, and actions before her seizure while identifying trends.

We established a chronological account of Mikayla's suffering, meticulously outlining the subtle nuances and changes in her behaviour and physical presentation that the medical professionals appeared to overlook. We then recorded her food intake, energy expenditure, and levels of carbohydrates, proteins, and fats. The programmes available to support this are exceptional, and this process has proven valuable, providing beneficial information.

The pattern was now clear to me. I printed the spreadsheet and showed it to every doctor—they didn't seem interested. They rolled their eyes at me when I attempted to explain the events and their relation to the seizures. That was the more courteous response. "Are you a doctor?" I was asked frequently. I replied no, but I knew how to collect and analyse data. Whether I was a doctor being questioned was more about asserting the power imbalance, and a clear one was in play.

Mikayla began seeing a psychologist to at least give it a go. The neurologists were adamant and refused to waver from the FND diagnosis, so we thought we might as well try therapy. What's the worst that could happen? However, the psychology sessions did not stop the tsunami of seizures; they just kept on coming.

Fortnightly psychological appointments led to the most bizarre suggestion: that her fear of vomiting was causing the seizures. I was speechless. What on earth is happening? Vomiting therapy was the final straw. After six months, the official diagnosis revealed that there was no apparent psychological trauma.

At this stage, I did not have a working theory on the cause of the seizures. The patterns I could generate on the spreadsheet should have been sufficient for any doctor to question the FND diagnosis and suggest that it might be incorrect. Well, that is what I thought would happen. I had no interest in discovering the medical cause; I was merely trying to help confirm that there was information to support questioning the FND diagnosis.

There was a pattern: use energy and end up seizing.

They ought to have listened.

There's no need to worry; she will grow out of it, were the standard responses. The seizures kept coming and were becoming increasingly intense, lasting longer, and occurring multiple times.

In preparation for our second home, I had the "hospital bag" ready to take to the ED: a phone, laptop, chargers, a calculator, a water bottle, and a set of clothes for Mikayla.

Before I left for the hospital, I would sit at home for a few moments and mentally prepare myself for the sterile scent of antiseptic, the doctors' indifference, and the neurology ward if they sent her back there again.

The ED doctors, efficient but distant, would conduct routine tests, provide the same weary reassurances, and send us home empty-handed. No plan, no support. The cycle repeated itself.

How can someone experience 21 emergency admissions without anyone questioning the diagnosis?

Every visit was yet another missed opportunity for a proper diagnosis, another chance to intervene and halt the relentless cascade of seizures. The accumulating medical bills and the emotional burden threatened to overwhelm us.

It wasn't merely our bills; I pleaded with the hospital regarding the costs to the medical system to appeal to their broader sense of responsibility for their profession. The ambulances, numerous callouts, the resuscitation needs, and the ICU. I can show you how to stop this, I said, but the initial diagnosis of FND seemed to loom over everything like a dark shadow.

We often felt unheard, and the system appeared designed to dismiss and disregard our concerns. The sensation of being gaslighted was a constant companion, a chilling awareness that our observations and fears were deliberately minimised or ignored. The repeated assurance that "everything was fine" in the face of mounting evidence to the contrary represented a form of emotional violence.

During every ED visit, I insisted that each doctor note, "Mother disagrees with the diagnosis," in her patient records. One doctor asked why, and I reiterated the question: Why? This way, if any legal proceedings arise, there will be evidence that I disagreed with your assessment. Even that didn't stop them from questioning themselves.

We continued to document everything. Every seizure, every ED visit, and every conversation with a doctor was meticulously recorded in a spiral notebook that symbolised our commitment. Each entry was a testament to our efforts to find answers, penetrate the medical fog, and secure the desperately needed treatment.

As the seizures increased, so too did the desperation. I cannot describe desperation except to say it was overwhelming. It felt like I was drowning in fear, while my frustration was less apparent than my fear. Desperation is debilitating, creating underlying emotional turmoil, stress, and a constant sense of urgency to act.

One night, in utter desperation, the doctors did not assist, and I felt entirely disempowered. I wrote to the Premier of NSW, the Minister for Health, local MPs, the HCCC, and a lawyer specialising in medical negligence. The only response came from the local MP, who informed me that I lived in a different catchment area and should contact the appropriate MP instead. Where was the help meant to be? There was nowhere to turn for assistance.

At this point, I realised I was on my own. I felt incredibly sad, but then I became defiant. If I were to make any change to this diagnosis, it was up to me and me alone. Bring it on, NSW Health; you have provoked this mother, and I will win this battle. I will protect my daughter even if you won't. But where do you start? And I had no idea where this journey would take me – the depths of despair, the unknown support I would receive, the un-denying beauty of connection.

Standing alone in the dark room, I dug deep, drew on every fibre of my being, and rationalised my abilities. I am intelligent; I can decipher this system and assess her health. But more importantly, my resolve surpasses the egos of a few doctors. I recalled telling the last two that they weren't God and to stop behaving like they were.

Ernest Hemingway once stated, "The hardest lesson I've had to learn as an adult is the relentless need to keep going, no matter how shattered I feel inside." I pressed on, lacking any concept of the path ahead, driven by an innate self-belief to protect my family. I have never shied away from exploring new avenues, but this journey was even more challenging.

One of the biggest problems was that Mikayla was seizing so frequently and felt unwell between seizures that it was impossible to get her to appointments in the private sector. When she experienced seizures, they occurred in public places or at work and lasted for extended periods. There was no option but to attend the emergency department at the public hospitals. What other choice was there? Leave her in public places? On the foreshore? With strangers? At work?

I learnt to advocate for my family, speak clearly and resolutely, demand answers, and refuse to be silenced. We documented everything, but rereading what we had written felt surreal. We continuously wondered if this had happened.

I asked, "Surely there is a ward for complex medical conditions?"

"No," was the answer. Really? The increasing frequency of seizures starkly highlighted the limitations of the healthcare system. It is ill-equipped to manage complex cases and often prioritises efficiency over patients' individual needs. Or I was being misled.

CHAPTER 3

TWENTY-ONE VISITS AND COUNTING

The flickering fluorescent lights of the emergency room became a familiar yet unwelcome part of our lives. Ambulances were called twenty-one times, though the number that arrived kept increasing. Only during the first one or two call-outs did a lone ambulance team attend. Each subsequent call brought two or three ambulances, with up to six paramedics attending. The fire and rescue services were present to ensure her safe transfer to the ambulance waiting outside for her.

We navigated the corridors twenty-one times, the sterile scent clinging to us like a second skin. Twenty-one times, we recounted our story: the same litany of symptoms, the exact frantic requests for help, the same spreadsheet but with new pages sticky-taped to the bottom, growing each month. It felt like a roll of the dice, a gamble with the medical professionals we encountered, a macabre game of emergency room visit roulette.

Naive optimism characterised the initial visits, a desperate clinging to hope that something would be different this time. This time, a doctor would listen. This time, they would conduct further tests to uncover the truth. This time, we wouldn't leave feeling more lost and bewildered than when we arrived. However, as the visits accumulated, optimism began to erode—a weary resignation set in, leading to a chilling acceptance of the system's indifference.

I honestly believed there was someone who could help. Was it because I did not explain it clearly? Was I not using the right words? What medical terms should I know?

My system involved preparing the physical items—the hospital work bag, clothes, and essentials for a long night. Then, I would mentally affirm myself, reminding myself that I am strong, intelligent, and capable of navigating this system. Doctors are merely human; they are not God. This is the notion I can cling to. Doctors are human; they are not invincible. I am intelligent, I love my daughter, and we have yet to explore everything. We are not finished.

I learned the system and tried to influence it. This was a significant task with walls and barriers I did not fully comprehend. I knew I was labelled as the bossy parent, which was evident through the gaslighting, but I didn't care until a diagnosis improved Mikayla's health. I started to use their systems against them, and then they turned, uniting their collective strength against us.

While some medical staff resisted, we encountered dedicated professionals who did their utmost within a flawed system. The missing pieces to the puzzle could have been hidden in the patient records. What was being said? What were the doctors' thoughts? How was our GP meant to decipher this if all he was getting were vague discharge papers?

Our ability to obtain Mikayla's patient records was hindered. Even when I cited legislation and health procedures, the majority steadfastly denied us access to them. "A doctor can read the notes to you, but you won't comprehend them," I was told. "You don't know me very well, but I'm confident I can." Was my reply.

What was everyone concealing? Why could we not obtain something as straightforward as her patient records? It felt like a conspiracy against us.

We subsequently printed the legislation and procedures to ensure Mikayla could access her patient records. We obtained the signed form, yet the patient records never materialised. Their suggestion of "normalcy" felt like a cruel joke, a mockery of our living hell.

Then, we discovered the procedures. I was researching, and some specific keyword searches quickly resulted in the top 10 Google list. These were public documents straight from the government's website.

Armed with printed copies of protocols labelled "MANDATORY", doctors and nurses would gaslight me, insisting they were merely "recommendations". "Let's test that in the coroner's court," I would retort, quickly adding, "Over my dead body will I ever allow you to get there to utter a pitiful 'sorry.

I endeavoured to keep meticulous records, desperate to impose order on the chaos. However, I lacked vital information hidden within the patient notes. This information would have been helpful for other doctors or the GP to whom they continually referred us. The discharge papers tell a tale of emptiness. For their effectiveness, you might as well leave with a Band-Aid and your name scrawled on paper.

I continued gathering information, carrying my thick binder overflowing with medical reports, lab results, detailed notes, and medical journals. Argh, the medical journals. I love research and dove deep into each Alice in Wonderland hole to find answers and information to provide clues. However, each time we presented this evidence, the binder felt like a useless shield against a relentless force. No one was interested in asking why I had it, what was in it, or whether there was anything special I had found. Of course, interesting information was in the folder – only the essential journals were printed.

The inconsistencies were staggering. One doctor would advise against doing anything, while another would inundate Mikayla with anti-epileptic medication. One doctor stated that another was on a fishing expedition. One would prescribe medication, and another would countermand the prescription.

One might suggest a gastro consultation, while another might dismiss it as absurd. We felt as though we were navigating a medical obstacle course designed to frustrate and exhaust us, a cruel game of "guess the diagnosis." But this wasn't about finding an alternate diagnosis – it was simply to treat FND.

The lack of coordination, conflicting opinions, and sheer indifference were bewildering and infuriating. Can you please decide? It was obvious that they couldn't decide how to treat FND. But hey, everybody—maybe it isn't FND! So, I tried a different tactic: Let's send her to a different ward.

"If you don't know what's happening, who oversees complex cases in this hospital? I asked nearly every doctor in the ED, but nobody had an answer. An illness must fall within the specialties; that's how you get admitted. Really? I'm not sure that even makes sense. Single-organ medicine is the issue," said another.

But what happens when you are uncertain about which organ is affected? Where do such patients turn? What about intricate medical conditions? There is no provision for such complexities. Turning away patients merely constitutes an evasion of responsibility.

Apart from the medical inconsistencies, there was also the emotional toll. The burden of uncertainty, persistent anxiety, and overwhelming sense of helplessness were invisible wounds, yet just as real as any physical ailment. But how does one overcome these?

As we pleaded with the doctors, presented evidence, and questioned diagnoses, they responded dismissively and, at times, even hostility toward our concerns. They accused me of being overly anxious, overly protective, and alarmist. We frequently experienced gaslighting, where our concerns were minimised and often invalidated, making advocacy more challenging. Anxiousness is not a singular emotion that defines me. Try something else from your playbook.

One night, Mikayla seized just as she was about to be discharged after eight hours in a triage bed. The reason was that there was nothing they could do – she has FND, remember! "She's going to seize," I said. "No, she isn't," the doctor replied. "Yes, she is," I insisted, "her heart rate is increasing." Three seconds later, as the numbers on the screen rose like those of a Wall Street trader, she was unconscious and seizing. The doctor looked at me in amazement. Amazed that I could predict my daughter's health. Amazed that I knew what was about to happen, and I wasn't a doctor. Probably all the above, but I didn't care that I was right – I cared that you could see what was happening.

Alarms were blaring, and the doctors did not believe she was unconscious. "We are merely testing to confirm her state of unconsciousness," was their comment as they yelled at her, squeezing her collarbone to see if she could tolerate the pain. "She is not responding," was the doctor's remark. "Yes, I know", I said.

MUM, PLEASE HELP ME

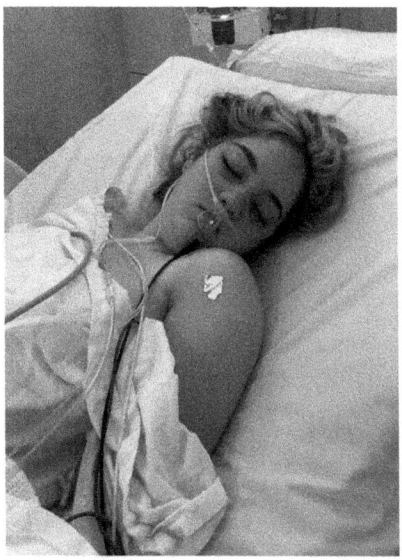

At that time, it was clear that they had not believed a single word that had been spoken to them for more than four months.

A part of me felt a slight sense of satisfaction—they had seen and experienced what we had been trying to convey. But English is my first language – what words would you like me to use?

Nevertheless, the power dynamics in the doctor-patient relationship remained starkly unbalanced. Our voices appeared to carry little weight, and the alleged expertise of the medical professionals swiftly overshadowed our concerns. Thus, we return to the same dynamic.

When the doctors felt I was asking too many questions, they would say, "This is Mikayla's illness; she needs to be in control." They used this line when Mikayla was unable to speak after just emerging from 14 seizures or had been unconscious for over 10 hours. What unconscionable behaviour!

Yes, she could open her eyes, yet she could not speak. She gazed at me with tears streaming down her face. You bastards, I know exactly what you are doing, and this will end. Mikayla and I had a code for when she needed my support, but it was evident that Mikayla could not speak coherently; nobody required a code to see the truth.

Our repeated experiences underscored considerable systemic failures, even though we encountered individuals who endeavoured to help. Each visit revealed the systemic shortcomings within healthcare:

- Lack of communication
- Inconsistent application of protocols
- Ignoring patient concerns
- The emotional and financial strain on families.

But I was trying to save my daughter and couldn't help others. It was overwhelming and all-consuming. I tried to analyse their behaviour: Why were they doing this? Why were they not helping?

I pointed out to the doctors that the cost to the health system would have been significantly less had they merely attempted to determine what was wrong with her. Not to state the obvious, but isn't it the intent, the objective, to get a patient out of the system, to stop them being sick, or at least to provide treatment? This approach is common in business: identifying and resolving the problem to prevent financial losses. The health resources we were using were adding up very quickly and did not appear likely to subside.

It served as a harrowing reminder that, despite advances in medical technology and knowledge, the human element—empathy, communication, and responsiveness—often remains tragically insufficient. We questioned whether we were doing enough. What were we overlooking? Were we somehow responsible for Mikayla's suffering by not simply accepting the diagnosis?

The constant barrage of conflicting information, the dismissive attitudes of certain medical professionals, and the overwhelming emotional toll had eroded our confidence. Doubt gnawed at our resolve, leading us to question our sanity and ability to advocate effectively. It takes significant resolve to be exposed to a continuous onslaught of "we are right" from professionals. At what stage does one begin to question their confidence?

Perhaps I had been overly confident those months ago. It was a rollercoaster of emotions. Yet despite the disappointment and frustration, each visit became a renewed opportunity to challenge the system's inertia, demand better care, and fight for Mikayla.

So, we persevered, seizure after seizure after seizure, ensuring that she was safe from the steel rails of the bed she was banging her head on, making sure there were enough pillows, and covering her with the sheets to maintain her dignity.

When I was newly divorced, I bought a leather lounge. It has witnessed tears of joy and sadness. It resides upstairs in my home, and aside from all its other responsibilities, it serves a unique purpose as the intervention lounge. Whenever family members wish to call an intervention or engage in a serious discussion, this is the lounge where we gather. Over the years, this lounge has listened to our fears and comforted us as we held one another and let our tears of joy or sadness flow.

This lounge inspired us to persevere. There were two occasions when I felt I couldn't go on. However, while sitting on my lounge in tears, Mikayla said, "Please, Mum, don't give up on me; you always have a plan."

It is an extraordinary place for gaining perspective, acquiring strength, and committing to persevere.

The roulette wheel kept spinning.

CHAPTER 4

THIRTY DIFFERENT DOCTORS

The twenty-one visits to the emergency room were merely the beginning. A symphony of confusion ensued. Each visit, although traumatic, provided little more than a reprieve, a fleeting moment of stability before the inevitable onslaught of seizures returned.

The initial diagnosis of FND, which felt unsettlingly conclusive, proved to be as fleeting and unreliable as the calm between the violent episodes. We were adrift in a sea of medical opinions, buffeted by contradictory diagnoses and ineffective treatments.

Thirty, to be precise. Thirty different doctors, each with their theories, tests, and prescriptions. It created a medical kaleidoscope that offered no clear picture, merely a perplexing array of colours and patterns. It was a shuffle of doctors, a relentless game of medical musical chairs, where I, the desperate parent, remained the sole constant in a changing landscape of so-called "expertise."

I possessed all the information, yet the doctors seldom sought my opinion. I implored every ED doctor to perform different tests. Their standard reply? "We must follow the protocols." I was at the heart of the information but was seldom consulted on what was and wasn't effective.

Once again, I implored each doctor to test differently, only to encounter the same response: "We must follow the protocols." Yes, but we know the standard tests yield nothing, so why are we still testing the obvious? Isn't that the definition of insanity: doing the same thing and expecting a different result?

But, reflecting on it, they weren't concerned about discovering a different diagnosis. They were comfortable with the status quo—carrying out the routine tests and checks. They provided comfort, stating there was nothing they could do. My position was clear: What you are doing isn't working—you need to do better. Look, my spreadsheets contain all the information.

Three doctors at the hospital recognised that more needed to be done to determine the cause of the seizures. One was an ED doctor who treated Mikayla on two separate occasions. The second was an ICU doctor who attended to her when she was unconscious for 22 hours. The third was a junior ED doctor who could see the underlying conditions. She listened, identified, and tried to act but was quickly stopped in her tracks.

Although they could see the evident patterns in the spreadsheet, I guided them through it; they were all constrained by the system and the protocols they had to follow. The brief moments of excitement when I believed there was a breakthrough turned out to be fleeting. Every path seemed to lead back to and be hindered by the FND diagnosis.

This system is utter madness. How can doctors not question, challenge, and advocate for patients when they see something amiss? Given that the admitting doctor has no long-term exposure to the patient, why is such significant authority granted to a single individual? Where is the system designed to support long-term complex cases or repeated admissions? Where is the team approach?

The irony I uncovered in this cycle of emergency presentations was that the reality in the hospital differs from the intended role of emergency doctors. The field of emergency medicine specialises in the prevention, diagnosis, and management of acute disorders, as stated by government health websites. Is having over 200 seizures, 21 times to ED, not classed as an acute problem? More importantly, if you cannot terminate, manage, or prevent the seizures, then maybe there is something else happening. Maybe that spreadsheet has valuable information.

Admission is determined based on the consulting specialist's agreement and the protocol's suitability. I experienced a gut-wrenching moment when I realised that the faith I had in the ED doctors was unrealistic. They could not help. Back to the intervention lounge we go, not for intervention but for comfort, security, and to find direction.

Could someone please explain why the "rules" limit ED doctors to the specialists they consult for certain conditions? I was informed that we must refer to neurologists for seizures.

Please don't – they are the issue. The neurologists were not paying attention and are fixated on a single diagnosis. They overlooked the deterioration. Look at the detailed graphs I prepared and printed, ready to present to anyone who cares.

The graphs are all colour-coded to clearly show the deterioration. The colours are purposely designed so that busy doctors can quickly analyse them. The four graphs represent all the reasons they should be considering.

However, nobody looked at my beautiful graphs. I was dismissed like a naughty child, and no other underlying causes were considered.

The seizures are the outcome; they are not the cause. I could feel the desperation rising.

The neurologists were unhelpful and fixated solely on FND. Several neurologists repeatedly advised us against calling an ambulance or seeking emergency services. They stated, "We can do nothing; there is no need to call an ambulance or come to the ED. It is psychological. Practice more mindfulness." In hindsight, knowing the correct diagnosis, had we followed these instructions, Mikayla could have died.

The hell she was enduring, apart from the seizures, was a constant wave of nausea when eating, lasting for hours, overnight and days. This left her bedridden for days due to fatigue and being unable to eat. Physically, she appeared grey, and her heart rate was elevated, even when walking to the bathroom. For most of the time, she was confined to the house. "Stay upstairs, Mum; I don't want to be alone."

On the days when she felt better and could go to work or out, we had risk management plans in place for every time she left the house. We structured simple mindfulness activities, such as taking the dog for a walk after conducting a risk assessment and attempting to balance independence with safety. With humour reminding Mikayla not to seize – you are doing mindfulness. But the humour didn't deny the reality of the mindfulness activities, resulting in the following clusters of seizures.

We wrote a note and attached it to our dog Meeka's collar so Mikayla could stroll gently—the phone rings. Strangers are helping; an ambulance has been called, they say. Note to self: A white note on a white dog is difficult to see. Next time, try yellow paper. Fortunately, the younger generation can access medical records on their iPhones.

That aside, Mikayla was experiencing seizures in public places, remaining unconscious for hours and failing to regain consciousness between seizures. Her unconsciousness would persist across shifts. Oh, you are still here; that was a typical comment. What would you like me to do with her? Put her in a wheelbarrow to take her home?

The absence of empathy in specific interactions made an already challenging experience even harder.

Mikayla seized at home. By this stage, nine months in, my working theory had identified there was a direct connection between low blood glucose and the seizures. But why was this happening? We still had no clear diagnosed cause—only my working theory. The ambulance paramedics witnessing blood glucose below 2, administered glucose for the first time, which helped.

She made it out of the house, not fully conscious, but there was no need for the fire and rescue to do that job today. Whoa—things are going remarkably well!

However, everything fell apart in the hospital. Eight hours before any treatment, she was deteriorating with high lactate levels, elevated ketones, blood glucose levels dropping, and beginning to seize once more. Can you help me? Fetch a doctor! My frustration is reaching a breaking point. Even when you are given information, clear medical information from the ambulance paramedics you still don't respond.

The specialist endocrinologist has been requested for a consultation. Her diagnosis is hypoglycaemic seizures caused by low blood glucose resulting from a gastrointestinal issue. Finally, the hospital caught up. I didn't even bring out the spreadsheet, she listened to Mikayla. I could have cried with relief; however, that relief was fleeting.

The gastro and endocrine teams began to argue over who would admit her, not out of a desire to take her in, but over who would fund the admission. The very first symptom Mikayla experienced, twelve months before her first seizure, was nausea while eating. This led her to lose 15 kilos in a short period. Investigations commenced, and although this symptom was not noted during her first two admissions, it quickly became part of her medical history. The initial symptom was thoroughly documented in the spreadsheet. But the nausea was also getting worse. However, the "experts" consistently overlooked it as irrelevant.

During this recent admission, the consulting gastroenterologist diagnosed constipation and advised Mikayla to visit the chemist. Although the endocrinologist was evident in her description, my silence did not reflect the anger building like a volcano ready to erupt. Incredible—could this get any worse?

As I looked at Mikayla, we both recognised the answer: we needed to leave. We have private appointments next week and should let the lawyers handle this. Knowing we could progress within the private system saved the arrogant doctor that day.

"Why aren't you using the private health system?" I was frequently asked. We are trying. We utilised the public system because she was experiencing seizures and was unconscious in public places or at work, requiring care during the days of and after the clusters of seizures. I had lost hope of guiding her to another specialty within the public system due to the referring protocols restricting the ED doctors and the barriers created by the neurologists. Nevertheless, I remained hopeful that the private system might offer more flexibility.

Alongside the public system, private appointments were often a lengthy organisational process, usually taking weeks, if not months, to secure. Ironically, we had to cancel some appointments because Mikayla was in the public system's hospital.

Five private doctors gradually pieced together the puzzle, each specialist contributing their part. Perhaps the most frustrating aspect of this medical odyssey was the lack of a cohesive plan. The absence of a centralised approach, a unified strategy, felt like a deliberate abandonment—a tacit admission of defeat by the medical profession. It wasn't until we took control through the private system that we were able to make progress, which took more than eleven months before we could make any headway.

The frustrating aspect is that the public system could have reached the same conclusion had doctors listened to the family, sought guidance, and not allowed the system to dictate the process for complex cases. But they didn't. They failed to take any of the actions that might have led to a diagnosis within months of the first seizure.

I appreciate that systems are vital, but I also question whether a human perspective can enhance a system rather than being used to suppress people. It is even worse when staff wield the system as a weapon and abuse their power.

We were left to navigate this medical labyrinth alone, without a guide, a map, or assurance of finding the exit. Without the support of our GP, who believed us, and two internal medicine specialists—one of whom insisted during our first visit that it was not FND—we would still be searching.

While I was able to research, locate, and digest medical journals, we still required doctors as professionals. It should embrace a multi-disciplinary approach, including family. The weight of this responsibility and the sheer enormity of the task often threatened to overwhelm us. The emotional toll was immense.

It is challenging to articulate how what started as a minor aspect of my mental capacity grew overwhelming. The perpetual uncertainty, countless appointments, and constant fear of another seizure drained us. We were ultra-vigilant – all the time.

The system seemed designed to frustrate and demoralise. Our lives became a cycle of hope and despair, a never-ending pursuit of elusive answers, and a relentless quest for assistance that often felt hopelessly out of reach. The system, meant to heal, was gradually destroying us.

Yet, throughout it all, Mikayla sustained our persistence, determination, and refusal to accept the status quo. We rallied around each other and found strength in numbers—it was all we had.

Our initial question frequently was, "Which specialist is on call?" Oh no, not him! Over time, it became all of them except for one. The mantra constantly repeated: to us, she already has a diagnosis.

The constant shuffle of doctors on duty was exhausting, disheartening, and often downright infuriating, yet it forged in us a strength and resilience we never realised we possessed. We used laughter, frequently misunderstood, as our own medicine. We uncovered the hidden strength of our family, the power of collective advocacy, and the importance of never backing down in the fight for the health and well-being of a loved one.

CHAPTER 5

THE TIMELINE

The timeline of events offers a comprehensive view of the journey through the public health system. This experience, characterised by a series of decisions, challenges, and varying perspectives, underscores the complexities of navigating healthcare services. By arranging these events in a methodical order, we understand how each moment contributed to the larger narrative—revealing the progress and setbacks and the evolving nature of our healthcare experience. The unfolding journey reflects both the strengths and limitations of the public health system as perceived through our lens.

MUM, PLEASE HELP ME

Mikayla's Timeline

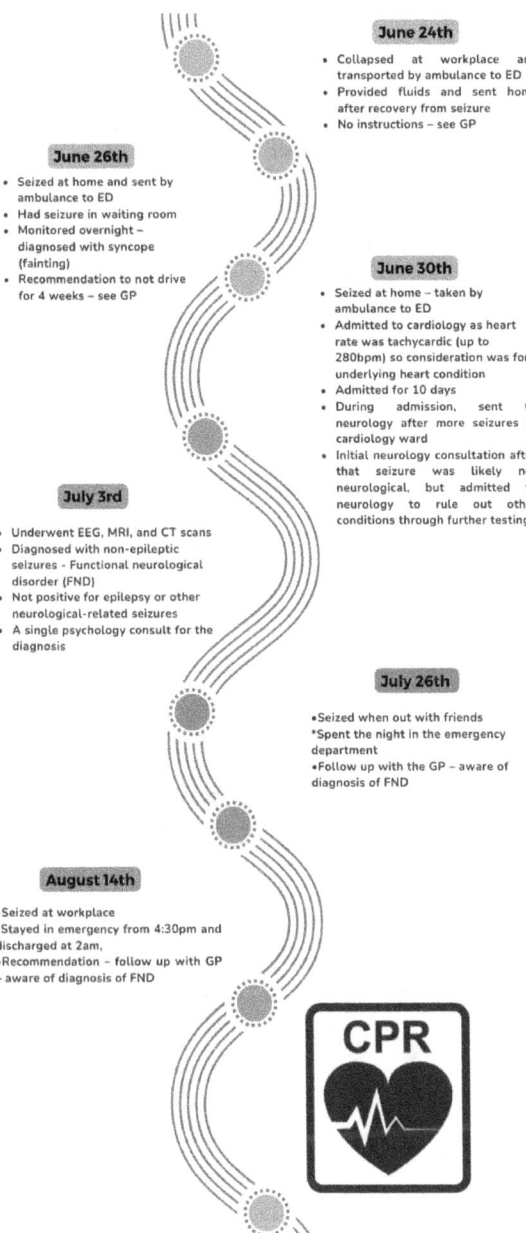

June 24th
- Collapsed at workplace and transported by ambulance to ED
- Provided fluids and sent home after recovery from seizure
- No instructions – see GP

June 26th
- Seized at home and sent by ambulance to ED
- Had seizure in waiting room
- Monitored overnight – diagnosed with syncope (fainting)
- Recommendation to not drive for 4 weeks – see GP

June 30th
- Seized at home – taken by ambulance to ED
- Admitted to cardiology as heart rate was tachycardic (up to 280bpm) so consideration was for underlying heart condition
- Admitted for 10 days
- During admission, sent to neurology after more seizures in cardiology ward
- Initial neurology consultation after that seizure was likely not neurological, but admitted to neurology to rule out other conditions through further testing

July 3rd
- Underwent EEG, MRI, and CT scans
- Diagnosed with non-epileptic seizures - Functional neurological disorder (FND)
- Not positive for epilepsy or other neurological-related seizures
- A single psychology consult for the diagnosis

July 26th
- Seized when out with friends
- Spent the night in the emergency department
- Follow up with the GP – aware of diagnosis of FND

August 14th
- Seized at workplace
- Stayed in emergency from 4:30pm and discharged at 2am.
- Recommendation – follow up with GP – aware of diagnosis of FND

September onwards

Aug 21st
- Seized at workplace
- Commenced CPR at work
- Seized at 9pm and discharged at 8am the following day
- Recommend follow up with GP - aware of FND diagnosis

Sept 6th
- Raised the issue of gastro problem
- Seized at work at 4pm - went by ambulance
- Attempted discharge at 8.30pm but had more seizures in front of doctor
- Doctor considered the seizures were epileptic
- Provided loading dose of Keppra (anto-epileptic medication) and 10mg of Medazalon
- Admitted neurology for 5 days

Sept 16th
- Seized at workplace
- Stayed in emergency from 4.50pm and discharged at 2am
- Recommendation - follow up with GP - aware of FND diagnosis

Sept 27th
- Seized at work at 8pm
- Discharged that night because the next day she had 5 day video and ECG monitoring and did not want to keep her

October
- 4 week gap between seizures as Mum put Mikayla in a wheelchair as there was an understanding of energy use causing seizures.

Oct 22nd
- Seized during walk with Meeka
- Administered Medazolan
- Started on dosage of another anti-epileptic medication
- Discharged next morning

Continued working out at gym because she was advised that is was epileptic seizures

MUM, PLEASE HELP ME

October onwards

Oct 24th
- Seized at gym - administered Medaz
- Had 14 seizures - admitted to ICU, had more seizures
- EEG monitoring
- Discharged from neurology on 29 October
- Advised by neurology to not call ambulance
- No tests were done to confirm epilepsy diagnosis
- Requested management plan - nothing provided
- The neurologists responded with "whatever Mikayla wanted to do and to practice mindfulness"

Nov 11th
- Seized at beach
- Admitted to ICU and went between there and neurology
- Approached neurologist to advise of GI issues
- Neurologist advised gastro issues do not cause seizures
- Administered 1000mg iron infusion as she was anaemic
- Discharged 19th Nov

Nov 29th
- Seized at work at 6pm - went by ambulance
- Discharged the next morning

Jan 1st
- Seized at home in the hallway at 9pm
- Administered 12mg of Medozepam
- Resuscitated in ED and continued to seize
- Discharged at 10am the next morning

Jan 2nd
- Seized at 11pm in her bedroom alone
- Paramedics estimated 1 hour before someone found her
- Paramedics administered Medaz - had 20 seizures
- Doctors thought it was epilepsy
- Given EEG on 3 Jan and admitted until admitted until afternoon of 3 January

Jan 28th
- King St McDonalds at 10-30pm
- Administered Medaz
- Admitted to neurology
- Discharged 30 Jan

Feb 10th
- Seized at home at 9.45pm after ice skating
- Given Medaz
- Discharged on 12 Feb - transferred to Westmead fro EEG testing
- Still thought it was epilepsy

KAREN PERKS

February onwards

Feb 15th
- During testing Mikayla stopped eating because she was nauseous
- Seizure detected was concluded to be epileptic
- Westmead confirmed FND diagnosis

Feb 21st
- After endoscopy and colonoscopy - seized while under sedation as she had fasted for 24 hours
- Admitted to ICU
- Monitoring overnight and released the following day

March 4th
- Seized after trampolining
- Given Medaz
- Discharged that night after 8pm

March 11th
- At this point Mikayla had continuous glucose monitoring
- Blood glucose was under 2 and it was advised to the paramedics where they administered glucose
- Ketones were high and glucose low
- Hospital knew her glucose was low and did not administer more glucose and she fell unconscious again

March 11
- Eventually administered glucose after 8 hours
- CT scan was done
- Endocrinologist diagnosed correctly
- Gastroenterologist diagnosed constipation.
- Discharged.

No More Seizures

Continued through private sector

CHAPTER 6

WHAT WILL WE DO?

I was frightened. During the initial admission in July, Mikayla asked how long it would take her to reclaim her life. I hesitated for too long to answer.

The reality was that it could be four months at best or possibly much longer. She sensed my hesitation and looked extremely sad. I realised we needed to play the long game, establishing a new norm until this passed. Let us begin with the good news.

With a brave voice concealing my fear of the "what ifs," I weighed the options. One possibility was that the doctors might find a diagnosis in the short term, and after four months, if there was no answer, we could take the long view. Regardless of the diagnosis, we must live with it. We cannot worry about what we do not know. I soon realised this was not as wonderful as I had hoped.

Beside her bed, we contemplated what the next four months might entail. Let us prepare for that period; if necessary, we can adjust to make this our new normal. We have faced this before, which feels like a lifetime ago when I was pregnant with Mikayla.

A virus affected my heart, and I was diagnosed with cardiomyopathy when Mikayla was six weeks old, with a prognosis of two years to live. Was this the beginning of Mikayla's illness now? There are numerous studies on the impact of a mother's ill health on her baby.

What was once standard, with three children under seven, was never the same again. Adapting our lives to accommodate an illness was not an issue; we will do it again.

But I remember the changes, the frustration, and the opportunities we missed, both as individuals and as a family. I was too ill to leave my bed, spending 18 hours a day there, alone in my room. Talking on the phone felt like a luxury, yet that simple act exhausted me. I recall the day I visited the hairdresser and slumped into the chair, lacking the strength to keep my body upright. I thought about how our lives had changed, and now I imagined how our futures would unfold again.

I remember my doctor at the ED, the two cardiac specialists who were my lifeline for 16 years, and the hospitals I stayed in. This was exemplary care. The standard of care I expected for Mikayla.

But with experience comes courage. Once again, I say, "Don't worry, kids—we've got this." Three steps ahead, I needed to ensure we were all adjusting at the same pace. Just because I remembered how to pivot and adapt doesn't mean they did. The experiences that Reece, Alana, and Mikayla formed during those early years when I was sick was their life – was their norm, so they didn't know what normal was, then or now.

Yet even I didn't know how far we would push the boundaries of routine over the next eighteen months. Watching your daughter's body fight against itself for hours is unexpected. Sweating from physical exhaustion and sleeping for days afterwards, it was heartbreaking to see her forced to accept this, even though we didn't.

The news was delivered. "If this is resolved quickly, let's consider four months." "Four months? It can't take that long; I have work," Mikayla replied, quickly realising that I had said "if resolved" too hastily, raising alarm bells. Her mind processed the alternative option I had yet to share with her, opening her up to the possibility of considering the other option – that it might take longer.

What will happen if we do not address her illness or establish a recovery plan? We need to implement long-term strategies. She was courageous; she asked how long it would take.

However long it takes was my reply.

Where do you begin? The house had practical aspects, but even something straightforward required planning, adjusting, and planning again. As the seizures continued to worsen, the plans we had implemented in July became inadequate by September. Reevaluate and plan again.

Consider what a functioning household might look like if Mikayla's health worsens. Despite outsourcing everything, we could scarcely, if ever, keep up with household responsibilities due to the demands of Mikayla's health. Walking in the door late at night, Meeka would gaze at us with those large, sorrowful eyes. Another walk was missed, and another day went by without playing with the other dogs. What are the options? This was the topic of discussion at the dinner table.

Our survival strategy was constantly being added to but, at a minimum, was:

1. Outsourced housework and pet care to focus on medical needs.
2. Created a spreadsheet to track symptoms and triggers.
3. Developed a flexible work plan to accommodate emergencies.

We engaged a dog walker. At the very least, Meeka was walked every Monday. Following instructions, Mikayla found a brief opportunity to practice more mindfulness and exercise. She would take Meeka for a short walk on another day when she wasn't in bed recovering. However, those walks would often send her back into the cycle of the ambulance to the emergency department for another night of horror.

We employed cleaners, lawn care services, and food delivery. Fortunately, we lived in a major regional area, making such delivery possible. When that didn't suffice, we ordered pre-made dinners. Everything was delivered, as there was no time to shop for food, clothing, or dog food. Nothing was off-limits if it couldn't be delivered—then onto the next retailer.

Work became the next challenge for Mikayla, Alana, and me. How does one explain to an employer that one is unsure when their staff member will be able to return to work? Fortunately, I could employ Mikayla a few hours a week to manage administrative tasks. Often, this was done from her bed, but who needs to go into an office to conduct research and data entry? I was flexible; if she felt lethargic, she could leave it, rest, and finish it the following day.

Her employer could also move Mikayla into administration for ten hours a week – a win-win for them both. Planning to rearrange a workplace required everyone to keep an open mind – and for the next eight months, Mikayla's bedroom served as both the office for my business and the administration office for her franchisee. Although it sounded ideal and was necessary, it also felt isolating. Work had become her sole social engagement; however, it also became a place where ambulance paramedics visited weekly or fortnightly whenever the new "seizure day" approached.

Meeting in the car park: Hi, how's it going? Have you been busy? Are we still on for Christmas lunch? The question of "what will we do?" wasn't just about household responsibilities but also about navigating life. I faced a much bigger question: What am I to do when Mikayla goes to the hospital if something goes bad?

Each time we visited the hospital; it was clear that medical assistance was being withheld. To avoid any misunderstanding, the neurologists and doctors in the emergency department emphasised that there was nothing they could or would do, nor was there any reason for us to be at the hospital, ensuring our unequivocal understanding of the situation.

I was frightened - again. One night, Mikayla was deteriorating, and I called the number to request a review, which the brochures stated would occur within 30 minutes. Three hours later, after multiple phone calls, the nurse finally arrived, saying they could do nothing. How do you know that? You didn't ask what the problem was, no consult, no discussion, no questions - nothing. The FND diagnosis is rearing its ugly head again.

After emailing the Premier, the Health Minister, and local MPs without receiving a response from their staff, I became concerned about my options if something went wrong, and I soon realised I needed a plan. That night, my worst fears appeared to be becoming a reality.

How do you persuade doctors to act? My more pressing concern was how to prevent them from harming her. I had two options: develop a media strategy or call the police to the hospital. Since implementing a media strategy takes time to action, contacting the police became my only option.

I wondered twice if this was a 000 call or a community policing number. How have we got to this place where I fear for my daughter's safety, in a place that is by design supposed to heal – not require protection from the police force.

In the morning, the patient advocate executive, NUM, and a third person arrive at Mikayla's bedside. Having been awake for 36 hours, I sit beside her with only coffee to sustain me. Although I have never undergone special forces training, being awake for 36 hours without food, in bright lighting, and with worries makes me feel like I have. There was no patient advocacy during that bedside meeting.

During another visit, the neurologist wished to send Mikayla to the ward in the middle of the night while she was still seizing. There is nothing wrong with her. There is nothing we can do.

That night, I contemplated chaining myself to her bed—desperate times call for desperate measures. I had their procedures in my folder, stapled together and organised alphabetically, ready to flip to the relevant page. The method for directing patients with certain conditions to specific wards was mandatory, and the neurology ward was not included in that procedure for sending a seizing patient.

At 8:30 a.m., the neurologist and I are arguing loudly about his intention to send Mikayla to the ward in the middle of the night. I will not allow you to sit in the coroner's court, offering a pitiful "I'm sorry" plea I loudly express to him. He claims there's no need to visit the hospital as we can do nothing. I look down; Mikayla is crying silent tears after emerging from the cluster of seizures, having overheard our conversation.

That was one of the lowest moments. We were alone, and nobody was coming with a life raft to help.

PART TWO

CHAPTER 7

THROUGH MIKAYLA'S EYES

I used to think of fear as a fleeting thing that would rise in the moment and then fade away. Now, fear feels like a shadow, always there, always looming. It's in the quiet moments when I'm alone with my thoughts. It's in how my heart races when I feel the slightest twitch or sensation in my body, wondering if it's a warning sign. My stomach knots whenever I think about the future because I have no idea what it looks like anymore.

I didn't realise how much of my life would be governed by fear, and how it would reshape everything I believed I knew about myself.

My first admission for neurology lasted seven of the 10 days. Seven days filled with endless tests and unanswered questions. Then, like a band-aid over a stab wound, the diagnosis of Functional Neurological Disorder (FND) was presented to us. I remember lying there in bed six, feeling exposed and vulnerable as the doctor delivered the news: "No driving for 12 months." No plan, no roadmap—just start with psychology and good luck.

Losing my ability to drive was one of the first cracks in my sense of self. I still remember the day my licence was suspended—it felt as though someone had stripped away my independence in an instant. Driving wasn't just about getting from A to B; it was about freedom. It represented late-night drives to clear my head, blasting my favourite songs, or simply being able to leave whenever I wanted.

Now, I couldn't even get to the supermarket without someone having to plan around me. I hated asking for help, feeling like I was holding people back, or being an inconvenience, but what choice did I have?

And then the doctors. God, the doctors…

I lost count of how many times they dismissed me, how many times they looked at my file with blank expressions and provided explanations that didn't make sense. I could feel the weight of their scepticism, the unspoken question lingering in the air: "Is she exaggerating? Is this real?"

Hearing the word 'psychosomatic' felt like a slap in the face. Fake. That's what they were implying—that I was making it up, that it was all in my head. I wanted to scream, to tell them they were wrong, but how do you argue with someone who has already decided not to believe you? How do you prove something that no one wishes to acknowledge? It wasn't just the dismissiveness that hurt; it was the way they stripped away my dignity, reducing me to a mere case study instead of a person.

And then there was that doctor. The one who waited until I was alone to ask invasive, humiliating questions. "How many men is your mum bringing home? Does this scare you?" she said, her words slicing through me. It felt as if she were trying to uncover some scandalous explanation for my seizures, something to fit her narrative. I felt cornered, as if a spotlight had been turned on me, exposing parts of my life that weren't even relevant. I wanted to disappear.

Throughout it all, my mum never wavered. When the doctors

doubted me, she didn't. When they dismissed me, she fought. She was my rock, the one who never allowed me to question the reality of my seizures. She stayed up late into the night, poring over medical books, searching for answers when the doctors couldn't—or wouldn't. I always teased her about that book, saying she should just write her own medical encyclopaedia by now. But deep down, it made me feel safe. Knowing that someone was in my corner, fighting for me, gave me strength.

She never allowed her crown to slip, even when I knew she was exhausted. She pushed for the right tests, found the doctors who would listen, and sat by my bedside every single day. Rain, shine, hail—it made no difference. Even when I begged her to go home, to rest, she wouldn't. She put her life on hold to ensure I had a life worth living. I could never repay her for that. She didn't just care for me; she reminded me, in every possible way, that I was worth fighting for.

Then there was my sister. She couldn't be there for every hospital admission, and I never expected her to be. She works full-time in a job that doesn't permit her to work from home, and I knew how much she had on her plate. Even when she wasn't physically present, she was my anchor.

She was the person I turned to when I needed to express myself. When I missed events and my sadness turned to tears, she was the one I called. When the frustration of losing my independence felt unbearable—when I couldn't drive, go to the beach without a risk plan, or simply live—she was the one who listened. She couldn't fix it, but she always found a way to comfort me.

I think a great deal about the day I spent at the gym. It's etched into my memory despite my hazy recollection of the events. I know I experienced a seizure there—multiple, in fact—and that multiple paramedics arrived. I recall flashes of light and fragments of sound.

Yet, the most vivid memory is the voice saying, "We're losing her." I'm uncertain whether I imagined it, or it really happened, but it doesn't matter. Those words haunt me.

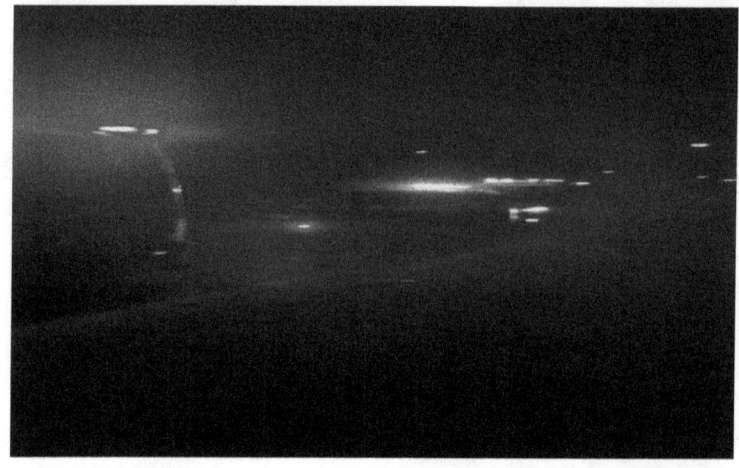

Ambulances lined up on major road to help Mikayla.

But that's all I have – fragments. My mum and sister have the complete picture. They remember everything: the moments leading up to it, how my body shut down, and the way they fought to ensure I was safe. They recall the fear, the chaos, the urgency. I only remember waking up to the aftermath – another hospital admission, further medical intervention, and more questions I couldn't answer.

It's unsettling to know that entire moments of my life exist solely in the memories of others. That my own story, my body's betrayal, includes experiences I wasn't even present for. I don't recall what led to it, only that it happened. But they do. I know there are specific moments, things that were said, and events that still weigh heavily on them.

Living in the aftermath of something you have no memory of is peculiar, yet you feel its weight through the people who experienced it. Their pain and fear are entirely real. Although I cannot recall those moments, the scars remain. And I bear that burden, too.

My sister was there that day. She remained calm, even though I knew she must have been terrified. She assisted the paramedics; she made decisions I couldn't. And when I woke up in the ICU, after what felt like an endless blur of seizures and fear, she was there once more. She always found a way to be present when it mattered most.

Sometimes, I wonder how she managed it all—balancing her job, her life, and me. My situation made things more challenging for her, but she never made me feel like I was too much. She never let me believe I was a burden, even when I felt like one. And that's the thing about my sister—she doesn't just make me feel loved; she makes me feel understood.

She's the person who knew when I needed a distraction, who could make me laugh when I thought I could no longer do so. She's the one who reminded me that I was still myself, even when I felt as if I'd lost myself in all the appointments, the medications, and the endless uncertainty.

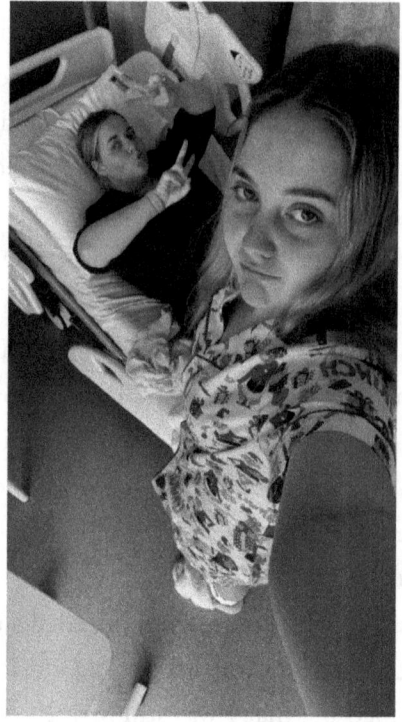

Always there for me.

But she wasn't the only one. When I woke up in the ICU, the expression on my mum's face conveyed everything I needed to understand. This wasn't like the previous times. It was worse. Seeing my sister there, her voice quivering as she informed me that Dad was flying down, struck me like a tonne of bricks.

Dad always kept up to date with the latest news; another seizure, another doctor, another hospital stay. Yet, there was always a sense of reassurance that things weren't urgent enough to require his immediate presence. This time it was different. Within 24 hours of being admitted to ICU, my dad was at my bedside.

He lived in another state, thousands of kilometres away, yet distance never prevented him from showing up when it mattered. He has his own life, just like everyone else, and his own responsibilities, but when I needed him, he was there. No hesitation, no second-guessing. Even when he couldn't physically be by my side, he ensured I never felt alone.

If I needed to talk, vent, or express my frustration about it all, he was just a phone call away. He never rushed me off the line or made me feel that my endless questions were burdensome. He listened, not to fix things because he knew he couldn't, but to let me know he was there.

When he walked into that hospital room, I felt a sense of relief I hadn't even realised I needed. He wasn't just another visitor; he was my dad. And no matter how old I was or how much had happened, his presence made me feel just a bit safer.

For the first time, I didn't feel the need to keep it all together. He was here, and for that moment, that was enough.

Support doesn't always arrive as you expect. At times, it's quiet reassurance. Other times, it's laughter—the kind that makes even the worst days bearable. My older brother—the one who's always ready with a tease or a joke, stepping on my toes just enough to make me roll my eyes but never enough to upset me.

He has an uncanny ability to lighten the heaviest moments, to walk into a room and make everyone laugh, even when the world seems to be crumbling. He visited when he could, and those visits always felt like a breath of fresh air. He never treated my situation like a tragedy; instead, he found the humour in it all.

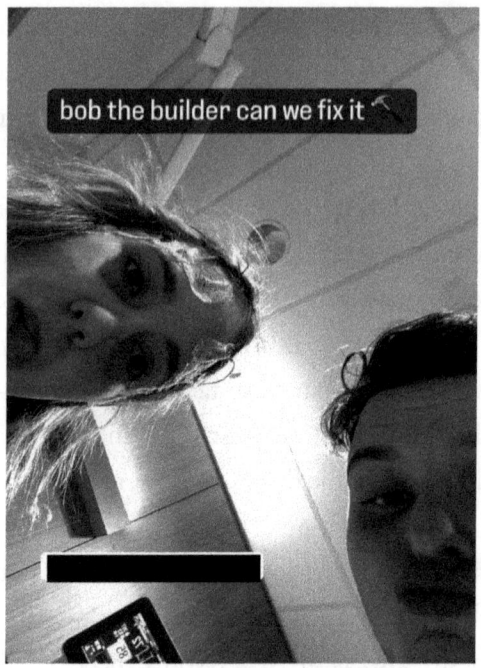

My brother, always the comedian.

Not in a dismissive way, but in a manner that reminded me it was okay to laugh, to find some joy, even amidst the chaos. It's as if being the class clown became his after-hours job—transforming hospital rooms into comedy clubs and discovering ways to make even the most challenging days bearable. He supported me in his way, demonstrating that sometimes a little humour is all you need to keep moving forward.

Beyond my family, others held me up. My friends, workmates and those closest to my heart became part of the support system I didn't know I needed. They were the ones who took the risk to go and do life with me despite the uncertainty. They didn't flinch when plans had to change, when I had a seizure, or when I needed help.

They stepped up, following my mum's plan, always knowing what to do if something happened. They didn't mind that hanging out might mean spending hours in a hospital room instead of at a café or that our time together often involved sitting in silence, in the darkness of a room, watching a film, or simply keeping me company while Mum took a break.

Some nights, after long shifts at work, they would still find the energy to visit, simply to sit with me for a while. Whether they came for a chat or brought dinner when the hospital food seemed too bland to bear, those moments reminded me that I wasn't forgotten and that I still existed beyond the four walls of my hospital room.

My last admission to a new hospital was for 22 days, and not once did they falter. They stayed by my side, turning a sterile hospital room into something that felt a little more like home. They decorated it, bringing life to it when everything felt so dark.

In those long, restless nights when sleep felt impossible, we would befriend the nurses, cracking jokes and finding moments of laughter in a place that often felt anything but life. They reminded me that I was still a person, not just a patient. And in a world that had taken so much from me, that meant everything.

Fear was a constant companion during those years, but so was love. That love, whether it came in the form of late-night research, a reassuring hand on mine, laughing at silly photos taken in moments of urgency, or a conversation that made me feel heard, was the only thing that kept me going. My network didn't just stand by me; they carried me through it all. Without them, I don't know how I would've made it.

But perhaps that's the essence of survival; it's never solely about enduring on your own. It's about the individuals who refuse to let you stumble, those who support you when your body, mind, and world seem to conspire against you. It's about the hands that reach for yours in the darkness, reminding you that no matter how burdensome it gets, you're never bearing it alone.

CHAPTER 8

THROUGH ALANA'S EYES

As the eldest daughter and middle child, I assumed responsibilities that were neither explicitly required nor openly discussed. No parent told me I needed to step into this role, but it was something I did, nonetheless. Following the divorce, my perspective changed. I was no longer just a sibling; I became the guide and support for my siblings, particularly Mikayla, during the critical years of adolescence.

But that is who I am – the nurturer. From 12 to 18, I faced the challenges of helping them discover themselves, not to copy my path but to encourage them to learn from their own experiences and mistakes. Yet, what about my growth? The truth is you don't finish growing—you evolve.

When Mikayla's seizures began, it coincided with one of the most challenging periods of my life. It had been two years since I had moved out of home, but somehow, I was still there for her, just as I had been before. Yes, she had two parents who remained involved, but I was her anchor in many ways; I was her sister. I had moved back home—not due to her seizures, but because I felt it necessary to be there.

MUM, PLEASE HELP ME

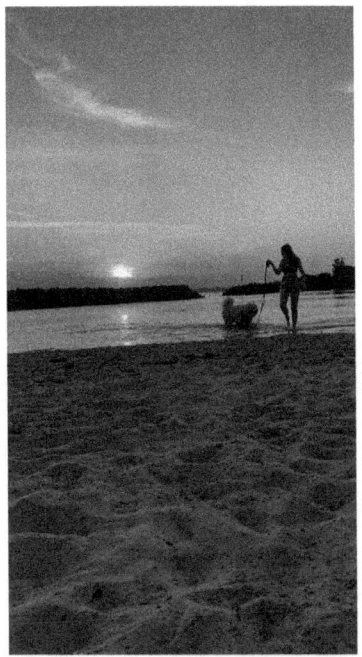

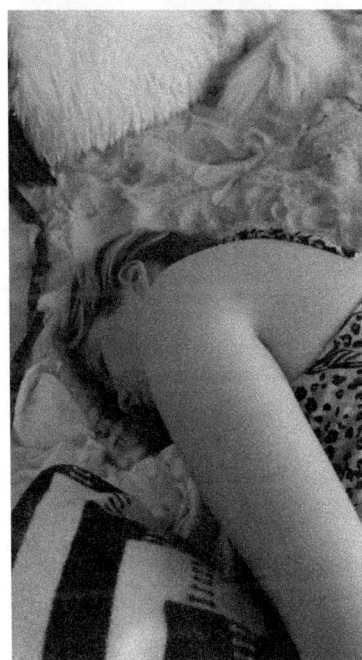

Mikayla at the beach

No one had truly prepared us for what seizures meant for a family. The first overwhelming thought that rushed through my mind was the fear that I wasn't doing enough, or worse, that I couldn't prevent what was happening. I was grappling with my issues, yet how could I ask for help from my mum when she was already focused on Mikayla's more urgent needs? I couldn't imagine burdening anyone else because Mikayla needed more help than I did.

I sought support from work and friends, using them as distractions, believing it would prevent my concerns from affecting their lives. It wasn't until I began seeing a psychologist—something I had never considered before, as I thought I was "fine", that I realised just how much I needed to process.

Every week, when Mikayla returned home after another seizure, she would look at me with those eyes full of hope and say, "I just want to be normal." I would struggle to explain that no one is truly "normal". How could I ease her pain? What could I do to support her and ensure she would be OK?

We discussed this as a family to make sure we all understood. With Mikayla sobbing, Mum getting frustrated, and me trying not to fall apart, I was always the one who could make everyone understand why we were feeling what emotion. That was my nurture: making sure Mikayla was heard and Mum was heard. If we weren't all on the same page to keep pushing, the fight for the diagnosis wouldn't have been worth it.

As the weeks passed, Mikayla's sense of independence further dwindled away. She pleaded with me to take her anywhere, just anywhere. I discussed with mum putting a management plan for the "just in case". I was tossing up whether to take her or not, I wanted her to be free of her own thoughts for just a minute and look for the future. I committed; I took her to the gym. It was a place where there were people everywhere so if I had split my attention from her, someone else could see her.

Nothing happened, no seizures, no paramedics, nothing. Mikayla and I drove home with the first real sight of happiness thinking, could this be it? Can they just go away?

So, we went back two days later, with the same management plan, the words coming out of Mikayla's mouth, "I'm fine, I'm going to another machine". I eased off just watching her to allow her to be in her own body.

I gazed into my own thoughts to what felt like a split second to looking around not seeing her anywhere. I called her phone, nothing. Immediately I sprinted around the gym. No, this can't be happening. I had seen her seize before so that wasn't an issue. But this was the first time doing it alone.

I found her, seizing on the bathroom floor. People asking if we are okay and just by the look on my face, they got help. I had the answers to every question the paramedics had like a textbook but eventually saying, "please help her". The text to mum was quickly responded with a phone call, I knew it was coming, she had no other choice but to trust me that I would make sure she's looked after.

Mikayla got taken by ambulance to which I told them there were more seizures coming, they took the chance against me without backup and left for the hospital. I eventually called mum when I got in the car and explained what happened and where they're taking her. I drove through the exit, around the corner, finding the ambulance pulled over, lights on. I circled with hesitance not knowing if my sister was in there by herself, or if there was coincidentally another person. Mum was still on the phone, to her panic, she was pushing me to stop and find out. I couldn't, I couldn't bring myself to look through the doors to make sure it wasn't my sister. The guilt, the sorrow, the worry. The thought of death was always surrounding with every seizure that occurred.

Eventually, I swallowed my pride and knocked on a closed ambulance door. It was her; they did stop as she had seized again. I was right. Mum and I were right the majority of the time, but what do we know, we're not doctors.

Mum and I buckled down, we must figure out a pattern. To our surprise we did, it was every Wednesday night. Seizure day. It was weekly, we made everyone aware, Mikayla wasn't allowed to be out for social events except for home or work on seizure day as we had to keep her safe.

We skipped a Wednesday; she didn't have a seizure. We pushed through the next few days with major caution, is this it? Is this what our life is going to be like? Not only for Mikayla, but for me? I had to make sure Mikayla didn't know this.

Those few days came to a quick halt with a seizure on a Monday, then Mondays were seizure days. I made sure I gave Mikayla one social outing a week avoiding the seizure days to keep her happy. So, we trialled places. However. Beach, seizure. City, seizure. Let's keep her home, seizure.

As the months passed, frustration continued to mount, particularly towards the doctors who appeared to dismiss Mikayla's concerns. Every visit to the Emergency Department felt like a futile exercise—no answers, no progress. The more familiar we became with the doctors and paramedics, the more disheartened we grew. Eventually, we stopped engaging, choosing instead to discharge ourselves as soon as Mikayla woke up.

Through it all, Mum remained Mikayla's staunchest advocate, yet I couldn't help but wonder why, as her sister, I wasn't allowed to argue on her behalf. Why did Mum have to bear that burden alone? It felt as though no one was truly listening to us, and no one was providing enough help. But if they weren't listening to Mum, what hope did I have.

Our lives became consumed with endless research—reading case studies, eliminating potential causes, questioning everything. The medical field had always been a place of trust for me, as doctors had helped me through surgery when I was just eight weeks old. But now, I was confronted with a frustrating reality: the arrogance of some in the medical field, unwilling to admit when they didn't have the answers, made the situation feel hopeless.

Determined to find a solution, Mum took matters into her own hands. We sought out compassionate doctors and explored natural remedies—all in the hope that someone, anyone, would listen. While some people thought we were mad, the true madness was how we began to see everything in shades of grey, realising that no one has all the answers.

What we came to understand is acknowledging that you don't know everything is far more powerful than pretending you do.

CHAPTER 9

THROUGH KAREN'S EYES

My eyes, which I looked through, were often open yet reluctant to absorb the view. They were moist from shedding silent tears. How had we ended up here, and how could I get us out of this? I was shaking, terrified, and yearning to wrap us all tightly in cotton wool.

I sat at my desk on a beautiful Monday morning, ready to join an online meeting with a new client. Two small, usually insignificant messages came through – they struck me, no, they battered against me. I couldn't breathe or gasp; what was happening? Every pent-up emotion - fear, anger, horror – erupted from me. Falling to the floor, I sobbed through the pain. How useless am I? Why couldn't I have resolved this more quickly? What a worthless mother I am.

The truth was, I couldn't bear to confront my reflection in the rear-view mirror. The woman I once was – strong, determined, endlessly capable – felt like a spectre. That morning, six months after the last seizure, I was sure of one thing: I had let everyone down.

That's what you call a panic attack, hitting like a freight train. It felt as though the walls of my life had closed in, trapping me in a suffocating labyrinth of inadequacy. My mind was a carousel of guilt and frustration. I couldn't stop replaying moments when I felt I had let my children down because I had failed to resolve Mikayla's health issue sooner.

So, it had caught me. I knew it would, and I had often been told it would. But this Monday morning, I was completely unaware that it would be that day. It was a relief. In my true warrior style, I shifted into action mode and confronted it head-on.

My parenting style was unique, shaped by the circumstances that necessitated it. I encouraged them to participate in as many activities as possible, facilitating their learning. While participating in sports and dance, they also prepared lunches, operated the washing machine, and looked after their siblings. We lived interstate and had limited support, so we managed everything ourselves. It wasn't simply a parenting style but a family approach we cultivated. We had an au pair when the children were young teenagers and utilised childcare from ages when Reece was three, Alana was ten months, and Mikayla was only three months old – all just babies... we fulfilled all our responsibilities but felt different. We were different.

A friend recently said, "If you don't belong, know this: perhaps you weren't meant to. Maybe you're being called to notice the doors only you can see and to step into your life fully and unapologetically." Our doors and experiences were precisely that—meant solely for us as a family. We needed the expertise of those doors to guide us through the next 18 months.

Failure was not a concept in our family. You cannot truly succeed unless you have attempted. Most importantly, we were a team; each member had a role and contributed. We were only as strong as our weakest team member, and no one was left behind. So, when Mikayla began to experience these seizures, no one hesitated to help her; it was simply what we did. We rallied as a team, a close-knit family, all prepared to do our utmost part.

Alana was confronting her life challenges, and she didn't need this. However, we don't run away from responsibility; we move towards it. Without hesitation, she committed herself to a new role with its associated responsibilities. In my mind, I would address Mikayla's health issue first, and then I could support Alana. Hang in there, love – it won't be long. Yet, it was a lengthy process: 18 months of spinning the wheel with doctors.

Alana became my wing-woman and backup. We dined and discussed hypotheses, new findings, and what's trending on Instagram and TikTok. Her new boyfriend entered our lives, embracing our chaos and sharing his knowledge of food and fitness.

We discovered videos portraying the experiences of individuals with FND seizures alongside those sharing their stories of misdiagnosis—young women from around the world. They expressed frustration with the medical profession, providing each other with support. What has happened to the medical world?

Reece has always been Reece. He will be a lawyer in a few months, and he views the world in black and white. He often brings me back to the facts; that's his approach. "Find the cause, Mum," he said in his direct, no-nonsense style. I am trying—oh my goodness, I am trying!"

Laughter has been our medicine throughout our lives. We treasure laughter, as it is the only way we can cope. However, when you laugh, only those within your inner circle—those in your group of confidants—genuinely understand your thoughts and can hear your fears and pains. We have learned that not everyone laughs at the same pace as we do, but laughter helps us cope, which is all that matters.

Holidays, business trips, and meetings were all cancelled like dominoes. Life was on pause, yet the days kept moving. Birthdays,

Christmas, New Year, Easter, Birthdays, Christmas, New Year, Easter. Seizure 1 … 2 … 3 … 4 …10 … 25… 40 … 62 … 87… 99…118 …140 …160… 200. Life came to a halt, and I became a part-time researcher.

The phrase haunted me: terrier dog. It was once a compliment uttered in awe by a professor colleague many years ago when I faced challenges with single-minded determination. I possess the ability to see solutions, realising that not everyone can do so. I was relentless back then, never giving up, no matter how complex the problem. Over the years, it became my identity. You could rely on me to dig deep and solve the unsolvable. But now, the strength that had defined me is gone. I am angry at myself for the dismissiveness I endured on the journey and the world for continuing to spin as if I were not already unravelling.

The dismissiveness I encountered along the way only served to stoke the fire. The doctors who dismissed my concerns, the well-meaning friends who told me that "the doctors are right," and the colleagues who subtly adjusted their expectations as if anticipating my decline – it hurt. But more than that, it made me stronger. Yet, in that quiet moment, as I sat on the floor, another question arose, cutting through my anger and tears: why us? Have we not already demonstrated our courage and resilience? What more could be asked of us? My family and I had weathered storms before, each one showcasing our strength and ability to endure. So, what was this latest test meant to teach us? What lesson lay concealed within the pain and uncertainty? It felt unjust, as if the universe-imposed challenges upon us without mercy or reason.

But deep down, I knew these questions weren't meant to be answered then. They were part of the struggle, serving as a reminder to look beyond the pain and find meaning in the journey. Perhaps this was a test not of strength but of faith—faith in us, one another, and the possibility of emerging stronger, wiser, more enlightened, and more connected.

That day, after the panic had subsided and my breathing had steadied, I resolved that although I might have felt useless at that moment, this was not who I was. My children deserved more than a mother drowning in self-pity. My family deserved a mother who fought her way back. My colleagues and clients deserved the tenacious individual they had come to rely on. But more than that, I deserved to believe in myself again.

The path to diagnosis had been gruelling, characterised by uncertainty and frustration. Yet, it also revealed something I hadn't fully grasped until that moment: the strength to endure wasn't something I had lost. It had merely been buried beneath the weight of my expectations. Now, it was time to dig deep and fight for myself, Mikayla, Alana, and Reece with the same determination I had always shown when advocating for others. I may not have all the answers yet, but I shan't give up. Terrier dogs never do.

CHAPTER 10

FAMILY, FRIENDS, AND NEIGHBOURS

We discovered our support network in surprising places. Navigating the healthcare system, especially when confronted with a misdiagnosis, felt lonely and isolating. The medical jargon, bureaucratic obstacles, and constant questioning of one's perceptions all contributed to a deep sense of isolation and helplessness.

However, our experience revealed the extraordinary nature of human connection, which can be subtle yet powerful. Love, support, practical assistance, and emotional validation are essential for survival. This lesson continues to resonate deeply, shaping our understanding of ourselves, our family, and our community.

We also learned about the importance of a support network. It is not something that simply materialises in times of crisis. It requires vulnerability and a willingness to seek help, which developed throughout Mikayla's journey. There were constants, but I love how our network grew larger and stronger than it had been in our previous lives. Neighbours, colleagues, and clients drew closer to our web through our vulnerability—staff who became confidants.

Initially, it was only immediate family. The family phone calls took place the following day when everyone was awake. We are a very close-knit family, but there was no urgency to wake anyone. "By the way," Mikayla was taken to hospital last night. "By the way," she went again. We didn't realise the journey we were embarking on; everything seemed fine, Mikayla was safe, we were in the hospital, she was being cared for... or so we believed.

In two weeks, daily phone calls with the family became routine. I was careful not to burden them with my pain, as it was their niece too. They were experiencing the journey and supporting our entire family, yet they had their own families to consider, and I didn't want them to feel overwhelmed by our sorrow. That wouldn't benefit anyone.

But when Mikayla was in ICU, unconscious for 22 hours, a wall of protection went up around us. The family were all there; we were shielded from the next round of pain. They filtered phone calls, updated the necessary people, and allowed me to sit silently beside her bed.

And then there are my friends. You truly understand who your friends are when long-term chronic illness becomes part of the family. I recall those late-night phone calls from an hour away, whether from Western Australia, Queensland, Victoria, or Tasmania, where my high-pitched voice could be heard. Meanwhile, they would promptly assess my level of stress. My country manager in the United Kingdom ensured the business kept moving, even though I was frequently awake in the UK time zone and could email in real-time. I remain grateful for her ability to read my mind.

Friends would send random text messages saying, "just checking in." It didn't have to be intense or require daily updates. The ten-second "thinking of you" messages were the most inspiring and uplifting words. There was nothing they could do but listen or ask, "Are you OK?"

These were memorable moments when close friends made last-minute changes to a long-standing catch-up that was being cancelled because I couldn't be far from Mikayla. "We are coming to you—stay where you are." And there they were, conveying their love and support through warm hugs.

But it wasn't just my circle; it was also Mikayla's and Alana's circle that offered support, sat, talked, and laughed at the silly photos. Nearly half the time, Mikayla was at work when the seizures occurred. Work was important as it provided a social outlet, and a sense of normality compared to her previous life. In consultation, her employer reduced her working hours to 10 a week and cut down her duties; however, Mikayla adored her workplace and friends.

Mikayla's work friends were aged between 16 and 22. We had a risk management plan in place to ensure everything was covered when she began experiencing clusters of seizures at work. These young individuals witnessed the events, assisted by calling ambulances, performing CPR, safeguarding Mikayla from customers, and relaying vital information to Alana or me upon arrival.

They meticulously documented the number of seizures, their duration, the intervals between each seizure, and their timing, ensuring everything was recorded accurately. They provided incredible support, both physically and emotionally. This exemplified the true essence of friendship, both within and outside the workplace. They would also visit the hospital to check in with Alana, see how she was faring, drop by her home, and watch films while Mikayla slept.

It was more difficult to hide the onslaught of seizures from our neighbours. We had moved into a townhouse complex three months earlier. With our busy lives, we often came and went throughout the day and night, and we hadn't taken the time to get to know anyone beyond the casual wave and shout of acquaintances' hellos.

Numerous ambulances and paramedics filled the long driveway while fire and rescue crews flashed lights like fireworks– they witnessed it all.

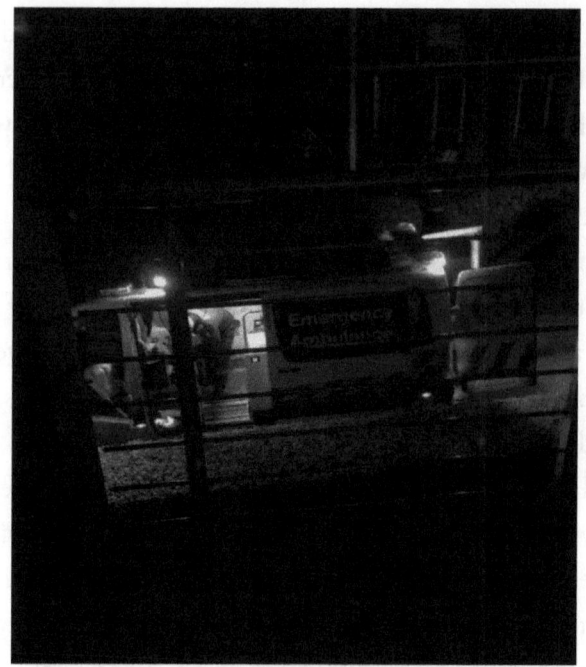

Ambulances were a common occurrence.

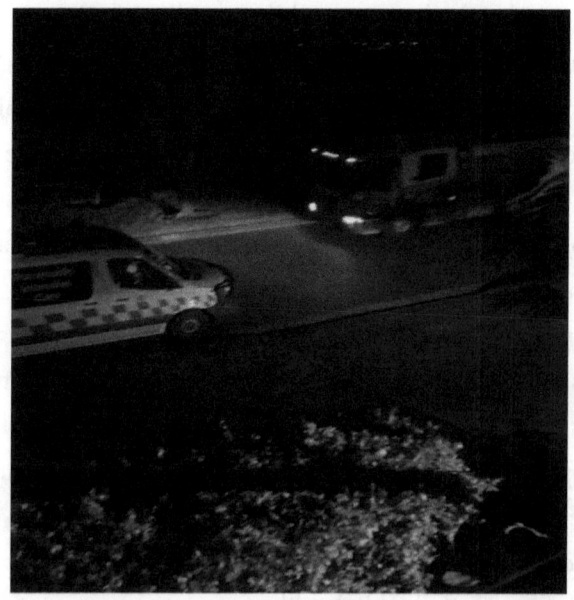

Accompanied by the fire and rescue to our home.

An ambulance blocking the driveway acts as a sudden introduction. Is everything alright? Can we help in any way? Does the dog need a walk?

These selfless gestures forged strong relationships that endured well beyond the forthcoming months. Their unexpected nature unveiled our neighbours as extraordinary individuals. They recognised the long days and nights spent in hospital, the emptiness in my eyes, Mikayla's weariness, and the lights that remained on throughout the night—receiving quick updates as I parked the car and stepped into the sunlight after a sleepless night. Nevertheless, I knew they were there, which was the most comforting thought. If I required anything, I knew they would do their utmost, and I am forever grateful and appreciative of that.

This experience taught us the true meaning of community. It is not merely about geographical proximity but encompasses shared experiences, mutual respect, and unconditional support. We witnessed the extraordinary capacity of human kindness to transcend personal boundaries, social structures, and geographical distances. We learned that acts of kindness, regardless of their size, can profoundly impact individuals facing immense challenges.

Support from your network is not just about their actions; it is also about the reassurance that they are there to help when needed. The unwavering support we received was crucial in our ability to cope with frustration, anger, and grief. It empowered us to find our voice and advocate for Mikayla, enabling us to secure the correct diagnosis and ultimately transform our experience into a catalyst for positive change.

PART THREE

CHAPTER 11

BALANCING MENTAL HEALTH WITH MANAGING HEALTH RISKS

For Mikayla, this journey involved far more than mere physical challenges. At 18, she enjoyed a vibrant, carefree life, embracing the independence and excitement of her age. She was full of plans, dreams, and energy. However, everything changed within two weeks, when she spent half the month in a hospital bed, struggling with the deep frustration and grief of losing her freedom.

Her mental health became precarious as she adapted to this new reality. The shift from a lively teenager to someone reliant on others was a significant adjustment. It wasn't just the physical limitations but also the isolation, loss of autonomy, and an overwhelming sense of injustice. We were very aware of the need to ensure her mental health remained intact.

Initially, she was without a driving licence for four weeks, which extended to 12 months. We didn't question the rationale behind this, as she was experiencing seizures every 10 to 14 days by that point. We discussed the reasons, the seriousness of the potential consequences, and the impact on other families and our own on the leather lounge—the intervention lounge. It was a sad but necessary discussion but deemed a "non-negotiable."

However, the loss was immense. Yet, it was not trauma and should not be confused with traumatic life experiences.

Through my work, I have gained experience with projects concerning social isolation and its effects on mental health. Furthermore, the most significant test of the impact of social isolation on mental health has been COVID-19, which we all recognise well.

We swiftly adapted and supported Mikayla as she sought ways to feel engaged, capable, and connected to the world beyond her bedroom. However, this was not without its challenges. Seizure clusters often accompanied an unpredictable routine, and every activity, no matter how small, required careful consideration and planning to ensure her safety.

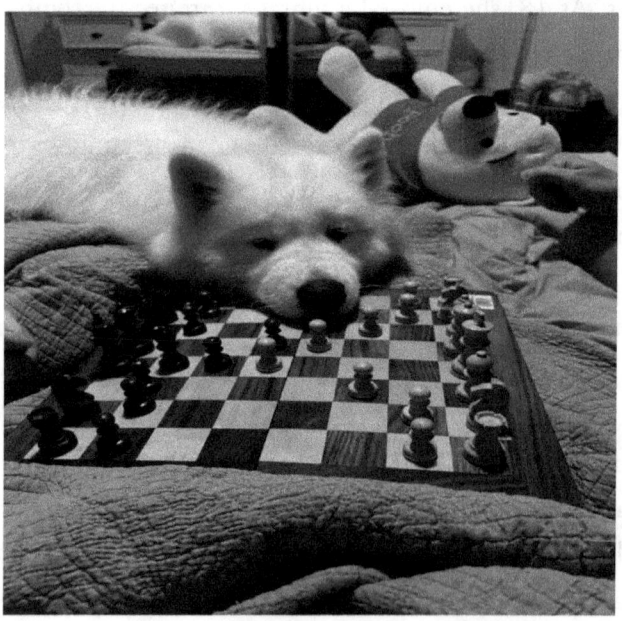

Meeka, your turn.

The key was balance. How could we support Mikayla in rebuilding her sense of self and autonomy while managing the real risks that her condition presents? It was a delicate dance, but we were committed wholeheartedly.

It wasn't just Mikayla that we were balancing; each family member also had to manage their work, activities, and mental health commitments. We developed a risk assessment and management plan for each activity to help us balance work, business, and personal obligations while caring for Mikayla. Achieving this required excellent communication and a guilt-free approach. The only person who felt guilt was Mikayla, as she worried that we were rearranging our lives to help and care for her. The reality was that we had, but it was never a question of not doing so. With an open mind, we had a solution for every obstacle that was thrown at us. So, we managed and succeeded in changing our lives to meet the challenges head-on.

It required significant reassurance to guide her to a stage where she felt no guilt. While this decreased over time, guilt would occasionally resurface when the frustration of lacking an alternative diagnosis month after month continued.

We operated seamlessly, like a well-oiled machine. We knew when I had meetings and work commitments, Alana aimed to go to the gym, and Reece needed to be at home to assist. Every detail was carefully arranged. On the surface, everything looked fine until the next round of seizures came.

We outsourced everything we couldn't manage—essentially, our lives. I cannot emphasise enough the importance of outsourcing or accepting help. It will spare you hours of self-punishment. You soon realise that you cannot do it all. Nothing feels normal when a family member is unwell. Acknowledging vulnerability is vital for maintaining your well-being.

With the planning, we all understood who to call first, who could go to the hospital first, and who would stay overnight. This was important for Mikayla's mental health as well; by being organised and prepared, we alleviated any guilt. She found comfort in knowing we could manage and balance our lives.

Prolonged periods of stress and frustration meant that the whole situation would eventually catch up with us all, though no one could predict when that would happen. We continued hoping we could stay ahead of the wave for a while before it crashed down on us, knocking us off our feet.

Our primary objective was to assist Mikayla in leaving the house. With her reduced duties of ten hours each week and her employer being flexible—permitting her to work from home if she felt too unwell to go into the store—it was a good balance. She frequently worked more than ten hours a week from her bed, and her employer valued and appreciated the extra hours. However, the ten hours were usually spread over multiple days to manage her workload. It was an arrangement that suited everyone.

Walking the dogs became a priority early on, even though outsourcing dog walking had been a deliberate decision to alleviate the pressure while determining the new "normal." Mikayla had always taken Meeka and Sass for walks, and this routine provided a dual benefit: it kept her active and instilled a sense of purpose.

It also aligned with the neurologists' mindfulness recommendations: to spend more time outdoors, increase her walking, and participate in exercise. Before long, we realised these recommendations were contributing to the problem.

One of the most significant breakthroughs in Mikayla's journey occurred when we discovered a direct link between her energy expenditure and the onset of seizures.

MUM, PLEASE HELP ME

We observed patterns emerging on days when Mikayla exerted herself physically. Even seemingly minor tasks, such as walking the dog, heightened the likelihood of seizures. Conversely, when her activity levels were low, seizures occurred less frequently. This realisation wasn't immediate, but when it did come, it was a sobering experience and, more importantly, a potential key to more effective management.

Armed with this information, we followed my sister's suggestion to keep Mikayla still, conserving her energy until the doctors were able to address the situation.

All my siblings and I were competitive athletes in our teens. Training multiple times a week and competing up to 40 times a year, we understood the interrelationship between food, energy, and bodily activities. We also knew what to eat to maximise our performance when our bodies were depleted.

With this insight in hand, we confidently chose to test the theory by markedly decreasing Mikayla's physical energy expenditure for a time and monitoring the effects. We deliberated on the available options for this, including how and what to measure.

I suggested hiring an electric wheelchair, and we all returned to the intervention lounge. Oops, maybe that was an extreme suggestion, but it has merits, so I threw it into the conversation.

When making decisions, we always ask ourselves: What is the worst thing that could happen, and what is the best thing that could happen? These are the only facts you need to consider. The worst thing that could happen is that it costs me money to hire the wheelchair, you don't use it, and we don't find out any new information. The best thing that could happen is that it makes a difference, and we have a clue what is happening.

The next day, we arranged for and hired an electric wheelchair for her use over the next three weeks. This wasn't an easy choice; Mikayla was initially hesitant, fearing the stigma associated with using a wheelchair. Well, honey, the options are:

1. stay in the house,
2. continue to be in hospital, or
3. use the wheelchair.

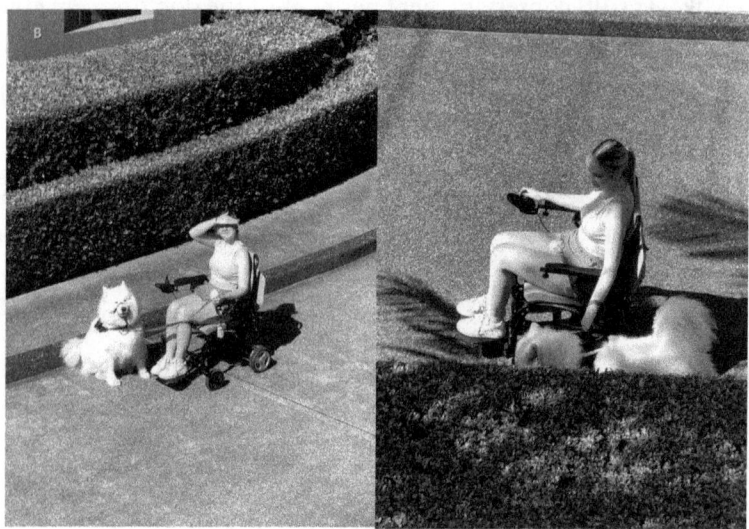

Wheelchair walking

We don't sugarcoat anything in our home—the facts are simply the facts. I explained that I needed her help to work this out. She chose the wheelchair and ended up enjoying her freedom, laughing while being outdoors. We framed it as an experiment, a chance to take control of her health and explore a new approach to managing her symptoms. And it was only three weeks.

The aim was clear: by conserving her energy, we hoped to disrupt the cycle of seizures. We encouraged her to rest as much as possible, and when she felt bored, the wheelchair enabled her to engage in activities without expending any energy reserves.

The results were astonishing. For 28 days, Mikayla experienced no seizures, marking the longest seizure-free period since her first seizure. Though initially a symbol of limitation, the wheelchair transformed into a powerful tool that restored her sense of stability and control over her health.

Her mental health was good, and she enjoyed the wheelchair. Speeding down the path and making Meeka run, I can still hear her laughter. But that remains a secret.

Understanding that her seizures were not entirely random but connected to something tangible, such as energy expenditure, gave her a renewed sense of hope. It also gave us a basis for examining the relationship between seizures and energy use.

This was my initial area of investigation, and since I am not a health professional, it was the only starting point for my research. However, over time, it did result in a decisive outcome.

The wheelchair experiment underscored the importance of thinking outside the box and being willing to adapt. It also highlighted how closely intertwined the body is. Just like a car—a machine—when one component fails, it creates a knock-on effect, emphasising the need for a holistic approach to a problem.

While this presents a simplified view of the human body, the doctors concentrated on a single organ, the brain, without recognising that other parts of the body contributed to the seizures. This has been the foundation of my entire argument since the initial diagnosis of FND—there was no consideration of physical contributors to the seizures. The gastroenterologists added fuel to not linking the underlying physical issues. Constantly saying – gastro issues do not cause seizures. My counter argument was – not singularly but your the doctor – make the connections.

There was no holistic approach to health; it concentrated solely on a single organ. What may be an effective method for a broken bone, stroke, or heart attack does not consider circumstances where an illness affects multiple organs.

This experience marked a pivotal moment in our approach to Mikayla's care. It taught us that, although frustrating, limitations could also serve as opportunities to rethink and rebuild. By acknowledging her body's needs and working within those constraints, we discovered ways to support her. Her mental health remained strong, with only slight declines during times when life became particularly challenging and frustrating, but nothing that we couldn't recover with laughter on the intervention lounge.

I shared this information with the doctors during my next visit to the hospital, excited about the new details to convey. Standing alongside the ED consultant and the on-call neurologist, with Mikayla in a resuscitation bed having just completed her eighth seizure—with number nine about to begin—I explained the results of the trial I conducted with the wheelchair. The neurologist might as well have said, "SO WHAT," as he turned away.

Dismissed as unimportant information, the ED doctor said nothing; however, I sensed he believed I was onto something when he later explained that the seizure protocol is to refer solely to neurology. Yet, it is not a neurological problem causing the seizures! It was evident that nobody was seeking the underlying causes of these seizures. And nobody was linking there were multiple organs at play here.

However, managing Mikayla's seizures and, consequently, her mental health remained our primary focus for the time being. We needed to address any risks she might encounter and be prepared. We started with the basics: plotting a specific route for Mikayla to walk. The route needed to be safe, manageable, and close enough to home so that we could locate her if necessary or see the ambulance if someone in the public called it first.

Fortunately, we live on a walking path and can see her from the balcony, although there are specific points where the trees obstruct the view. We didn't mention it to her for a little while. We considered every detail, including the time of day, to ensure other people were also out and about. One of us could have accompanied Mikayla, but she felt she was losing her independence and being watched over constantly, so we held our breath and let her venture out independently.

We considered the amount of energy she had expended on the previous day and the current one, as well as the quantity of food she had consumed. We attached a note with emergency contact details to Meeka's collar to enhance safety. It seemed like a clever idea—until we realised our oversight when Mikayla had a seizure during a walk late one afternoon.

The white paper was almost invisible against Meeka's white fur, so nobody noticed the note. We learned a lesson, and we adapted by using bright yellow paper for future outings. It was a minor change, but it highlighted the importance of attending to even the smallest detail and considering various scenarios.

Mikayla's friends became an essential part of her support network. We recognised that nurturing her social connections was crucial for her mental health. Her friends served as her emotional anchors and allies in safeguarding her well-being and safety.

To facilitate this, we provided them with all the necessary contact details and clear guidance on what to do if Mikayla needed assistance whilst out. Everyone had a role to play, and this coordination instilled in Mikayla the confidence to venture out, knowing that a network of people who cared about her wellbeing was supporting her. It also reassured her friends on how to respond when Mikayla was distressed or seizing.

This system assured us, her family, that she was not alone. Our collaboration with her friends established a safety net that allowed Mikayla to explore her independence within carefully defined boundaries. It also safeguarded her friends in what were often frightening situations for them—but they were amazing.

While managing risks was essential, the aim was empowerment. Once more, we wanted Mikayla to feel capable and in control of her life. This involved focusing on activities she could enjoy and benefit from without physically overwhelming her or adding to her stress.

Mikayla's journey was a valuable learning experience for us all. We learned the importance of being adaptable and creative in addressing her needs. Every setback—such as the white paper on Meeka—taught us something new about how to support her better.

One of the major lessons was recognising that risk mitigation doesn't equate to eliminating all risks. It involves managing them thoughtfully to create opportunities for growth and connection. Mikayla's mental health improved not because we shielded her from every potential challenge, but because we discovered ways to help her navigate them safely and confidently.

We laughed at all the setbacks: the white paper, parking the wheelchair in the garage, and the fire trucks in our driveway. We found the tiniest bit of humour in everything. Humour does not lessen the seriousness of what is happening, but for us, it brings a balance to the horror.

Clear communication was the backbone of our approach. Open and honest conversations were essential, whether coordinating with her friends, planning activities, or simply checking in with Mikayla about her feelings. We often used the intervention lounge to check in with

Mikayla, ensuring she felt heard and understood, which gave her the emotional strength to face her challenges. We also invited Mikayla's friends to the intervention lounge, recognising their significance and acknowledging the importance of checking in with them about their feelings.

The intervention lounge has had significant workouts over the past few years, but it has also held us tightly and grounded. We love the space it gives us to be honest with each other and open about how we are feeling. We even have our little part of the lounge where we like to position ourselves, ready for conversations. We highly recommend everyone have one of these safe places to be kind and honest.

CHAPTER 12

PARENTAL INTUITION AND RESEARCH

The initial diagnosis, delivered with the practiced assurance of a seasoned neurologist, struck with the force of a hammer blow: FND. This term resonated with fear and uncertainty, encapsulating all the terrifying unknowns swirling around the increasingly frequent seizures.

But even as we grappled with the enormity of the diagnosis, a small seed of doubt began to surface. Something didn't quite fit. The seizures, while undeniably alarming, but did not align neatly with the typical patterns described in the medical literature I desperately consumed during sleepless nights.

The frequency of the seizures began with a single episode, peaking at over 15 seizures lasting up to 15 minutes each, with unconsciousness averaging between 10 and 15 hours and occasionally reaching 22 hours. This was not typical for FND, according to the literature. The variations in presentation and the absence of any discernible trigger all felt rather unusual. The prescribed medication had failed to resolve the issue, having no effect whatsoever—neither the cardiac medication, anti-seizure medication, nor psychiatric medication worked to halt or even reduce the seizures.

There were still those terrifying moments when she would roll her eyes, her heart racing, and then she would seize. The only pattern was the rapid heart rate—a sign she was about to seize. Fear was a constant companion, a chilling undercurrent to our daily lives.

This was not merely about the seizures but about the lack of a thorough investigation. I felt as though we were being hurried through a standardised process, with a diagnosis quickly assigned without a comprehensive exploration of alternative possibilities. The sensation of being unheard, with our concerns brushed aside with a wave of the hand and a reassuring, though unconvincing, pat on the back, gnawed at me.

Thus began our parallel journey. One unfolded within the sterile confines of the hospital and doctors' rooms, while the other took place in the digital realm of online medical journals and forums. My days were a blur of attempting to keep the business running whilst I spent my nights poring over medical texts, comparing symptoms, and searching for alternative explanations.

I became a self-taught expert, armed with printouts of research papers and detailed charts tracking every seizure and medication dosage—or at least a novice expert. I was putting the pieces together in the puzzle.

Mikayla and Alana conducted their own research examining social media platforms such as Instagram, TikTok, and Facebook. There were numerous sites, all with similar issues – misdiagnosis, FND, and seizures — affecting not just Australia but also the world. Predominantly women who had been overlooked or misdiagnosed. However, for our family, we all reached the same conclusion: we firmly believed it was not FND.

My favourite has always been the Mayo Clinic. The intelligence of the people who work there is remarkable, with many medical journals written by specialists from the Mayo Clinic. Although it is headquartered in the United States, they have centres around the world. I looked — but not in Australia. Another question I had on my list was: why is the Mayo Clinic not in Australia? We obviously face the same problems as the rest of the world.

Then there were the international medical journals I gathered, which provided evidence from around the globe regarding the various potential causes of Mikayla's seizures and the reasons why they could not or would not be FND.

My research was not merely a desperate attempt to find answers; it served as a way to regain control in a situation where we felt utterly powerless. Each article I read inspired me. There were so many that offered explanations of alternative physical causes of seizures. I kept asking myself, why was FND diagnosed as the only option so early on?

What was the agenda in diagnosing FND? Then I became cynical - does it generate more funding for the hospital? It is a trending diagnosis. There must be a reason the neurologists remained so single-minded in their opinion. Only the patient notes could provide any insight into their thinking, the opinions, and the narrow-mindedness to not consider all the information that I found so easily in medical journals, despite not being a doctor, as they kept reminding me.

The medical journals are now printed out and safe in my folder or saved in the folders on my computer. But both places were always with me, and by default, I was always in the hospital with them. Somebody, anybody, just needed to listen; I wasn't waiting for them to ask.

I wasn't alone. Other parents and families shared similar stories: initial misdiagnoses coupled with dismissed concerns and a frustrating battle to receive appropriate care. Although our health problems varied, as did the states and countries, the treatment, non-treatment, or incorrect diagnosis of complex health conditions was similar – this reflects an international issue. A professional issue.

The feeling of isolation was overwhelming. We felt alone in our struggle. Our family and friends, while supportive, found it difficult to understand the depth of our frustration and the relentless weight of our anxiety. At first, their well-meaning words, "Just trust the doctors," felt like a slap in the face.

We wanted to trust the doctors, and we needed to. However, the overwhelming evidence contradicted the diagnosis, undermining our reasons for trusting them. We needed to understand why Mikayla was suffering, and that knowledge could not come through blind faith.

While often a source of misinformation, the internet has proven to be a vital tool in our quest for answers. We meticulously vetted the information we uncovered, cross-referencing multiple sources. We compiled folders of articles, studies, and anecdotal evidence that illuminated the possibility of alternative diagnoses—diagnoses that better accounted for the unique characteristics of not only Mikayla's seizures but also other physiological causes of seizures, as we sought to understand what was happening with her body.

The painstaking research process was emotionally draining, yet it was also strangely empowering. The more I learned, the more confident I became in our ability to challenge the initial diagnosis. We were no longer passive recipients of medical care; we had transformed into active participants in Mikayla's treatment, assuming the role of our own advocates. This shift in mindset was crucial. The initial sense of helplessness gradually gave way to a quiet determination and a resolute focus on uncovering the truth.

However, this research also posed a challenge. The sheer volume of information was overwhelming and necessitated a methodical approach. Once again, I would use humour to joke about my part-time and unpaid role. Sifting through numerous studies, navigating conflicting opinions, and identifying relevant research demanded immense time and effort.

The medical terminology was often dense, yet it became comprehensible when read slowly and in fragments. Fortunately, my work frequently involved unpacking complex concepts, including medical ones, which allowed me to apply my analytical skills and meticulously examine every relevant medical journal.

This self-directed research not only focused on discovering alternative diagnoses but also aimed to explore the complexities of the medical system, the shortcomings of current diagnostic tools, and the potential for human error.

This also meant that my mind operated for 18 hours a day, often with limited sleep. The physical and emotional toll was mounting. The persistent worry, the sleepless nights, and the never-ending research all contributed to a feeling of exhaustion and burnout.

We had to be extremely mindful of our well-being, ensuring that we took breaks, sought support from our loved ones, and prioritised our mental health. We learned that advocacy is a marathon, not a sprint, and that maintaining our well-being was crucial to effectively advocate for Mikayla.

This was not merely a collection of medical data but was fuelled by parental intuition, an instinctive understanding of Mikayla's needs, and a relentless pursuit of truth. It embodied unwavering hope, a refusal to accept a fundamentally incorrect diagnosis, and a powerful demonstration of the strength and resilience within our hearts.

Initially small and delicate, the seeds of doubt had taken root and were blossoming into a formidable force. The battle had only just begun, yet we were armed with more than mere hope; we were equipped with evidence. We were ready to fight.

MUM, PLEASE HELP ME

One night in February, eight months after the first seizure, I watched a TEDx talk. The American cardiologists applying artificial intelligence (AI) to diagnose complex conditions that had previously remained unresolved in patients who had consulted 20 to 30 doctors.

I had not considered applying AI to our situation, although I had confidently used it in other areas. In the following months, I short-listed the two conditions contributing to the seizures. I figured out how to apply AI effectively to support medical diagnoses for Mikayla.

CHAPTER 13

AI AND MEDICAL DIAGNOSIS – IS THIS THE FUTURE?

The field of medicine is undergoing a significant transformation, with AI at its core. Diagnosing illnesses has long been a human endeavour, relying on the expertise and intuition of clinicians for centuries. Today, AI is at the forefront of this evolution, becoming a partner in diagnosis, capable of analysing complex data and uncovering patterns that humans might overlook.

AI in healthcare employs computers to analyse medical data. It assists doctors in identifying patterns that may be overlooked in traditional diagnoses. This statement alone is sufficient to create a divide within the medical profession regarding the use of AI in diagnosis.

Why would doctors and anyone in the medical profession be dismissiveness of AI technological advancements? Technological advancements have been the whole backbone of the medical profession since the industrial revolution, and if not before. We could not live without any of these but there was also a time when these diagnostic devices were new to the profession and what we now take for granted as standard medical devices and diagnostics.

- X Ray Machines
- MRI
- Ultrasounds
- Heart Monitors
- CT Scanners (Computed Tomography)
- PET Scanners (Positron Emission Tomography)
- Endoscopes
- Echocardiograms
- Electroencephalogram (EEG)
- Genetic Testing
- Cryotherapy
- Robotic Surgery
- Laser Surgery
- 3D Printing in Medicine
- Wearable Health Monitors
- Artificial Organs
- Immunotherapy
- Stem Cell Therapy
- Smart Inhalers

Such as AI is now. New to the world – new to the medical profession. As those medical devices once were.

But how far can AI progress? Could it eventually surpass human doctors in terms of accuracy? Or is the true potential realised through collaboration, where machines and humans work together to achieve results that neither could accomplish alone?

AI is no longer a distant concept in healthcare; it has arrived and is making significant strides. From advanced imaging analysis to predictive algorithms, AI applications are transforming the diagnostic process.

Traditionally, diagnosis has entailed gathering patient histories, conducting physical examinations, and interpreting tests—a process that often relied on the clinician's training and experience. While effective, it is not free from human error or time constraints. Enter AI, with its ability to process vast datasets, identify subtle correlations, and deliver evidence-based insights at unprecedented levels and speeds.

AI systems are already making significant contributions in fields such as radiology, dermatology, and pathology. For instance, in some countries, deep learning algorithms can detect anomalies in imaging scans, including tumours or fractures, with an accuracy that rivals that of expert physicians. Meanwhile, natural language processing (NLP) tools analyse electronic health records to flag potential issues or propose diagnoses based on patients' medical histories.

The rise of AI is not merely a matter of technological novelty; it addresses several critical challenges in healthcare, such as speed, efficiency, accuracy, accessibility, and personalisation. Each of these critical challenges in healthcare remains unresolved. Why are we hesitating?

There are sick people all over Australia, particularly in regional and remote areas, within underprivileged socio-economic groups, including women and children – why are we hesitating? Additionally, there is the ongoing debate about the costs of visiting GPs and specialists – why are we not wholeheartedly embracing modern technology?

Grasping the advantages of AI in medical diagnosis should excite many. This is not a field we can overlook, not just for the health of the citizens of our nation, but also for the innovation and economic opportunities it presents for our country.

At a very high level, these advantages could potentially achieve:

1. Speed and efficiency

AI can analyse data in seconds, minimising the time required for diagnoses. In time-sensitive situations, such as identifying strokes or cardiac issues, this speed can make the difference between life and death.

2. Accuracy and consistency

Even the most experienced clinicians can suffer from fatigue and occasional oversights. In contrast, AI systems provide consistent results, ensuring that no detail is missed.

3. Accessibility

In remote or underserved regions, access to specialised care is often limited. AI-powered diagnostic tools, deployed via mobile devices or standalone systems, provide expertise to these areas, bridging the gap between patients and their healthcare providers. They can also support GPs by accelerating the diagnostic process.

4. Personalisation

By analysing genetic, environmental, and lifestyle factors, AI enhances precision medicine by offering tailored insights that surpass traditional diagnostic methods.

CHALLENGES AND ETHICAL CONSIDERATIONS

Despite its potential, AI in diagnosis has its challenges. However, these challenges are not reasons to use AI; they are challenges we need to understand and mitigate any risks. These challenges are not boulders in our way—they are warning signs. Warning signs are just that—warnings to have a higher consciousness. All these challenges are just that—warnings to be conscious of and address.

1. Data privacy and security
AI systems rely on extensive datasets, often containing sensitive patient information. Safeguarding this data from breaches and maintaining ethical standards and usage is essential.

2. Bias in algorithms
AI models are only as unbiased as the data on which they are trained. If the training data lacks diversity or reflects existing inequities, the AI may perpetuate or even exacerbate disparities in healthcare.

3. Lack of human intuition
AI excels in pattern recognition but lacks the intuition and contextual understanding that a human clinician possesses. It cannot comprehend the subtleties of a patient's lived experience or emotional nuances.

4. Risk of over-reliance
There is a risk that clinicians may become overly reliant on AI, which could undermine their diagnostic skills. AI should enhance human expertise, not supplant it.

AI is already demonstrating its value in clinical settings

In certain parts of the world, AI is being utilised in several areas—areas that we should be enthusiastic about. This demonstrates how AI enhances diagnostic capabilities, making healthcare more efficient and accurate. In radiology, cardiology, neurology, dermatology and pathology.

The most promising vision of AI in diagnosis lies in collaboration rather than replacement. While AI can process and analyse data on a scale unmatched by humans, clinicians offer a level of empathy, intuition, and holistic understanding that machines cannot replicate.

Doctors and AI collaborating. Such inspiration – such potential for saving lives.

AI acts as a second opinion: Algorithms identify potential issues, providing clinicians with enhanced insights to aid their decision-making.

AI enhances training: By simulating rare or complex scenarios, AI supports the training of the next generation of doctors.

AI facilitates early detection: By recognising initial warning signs, AI empowers clinicians to intervene before conditions escalate significantly.

The question is not whether AI will shape the future of diagnosis—it already does. The real question is how we can responsibly and effectively harness its capabilities and potential. In an ideal future, AI will not replace doctors but empower them. It will relieve the burden of routine tasks, allowing clinicians to concentrate on complex cases and patient relationships. AI will also democratise access to high-quality care, ensuring that even the most remote or underserved populations benefit from technological advancements.

Nevertheless, this future hinges on tackling the challenges of bias, privacy, and overdependence. It requires that AI continues to augment human capabilities rather than diminish them.

AI and medical diagnosis signify a partnership with remarkable potential. It suggests a future where technology and human ingenuity collaborate to enhance health outcomes and deepen the understanding of medical practice.

While AI will never fully replace the clinician's role, it can fundamentally transform it. Together, humans and AI can achieve what neither could accomplish alone: a quicker, more precise, and more accessible healthcare system.

Our goal wasn't to substitute the clinician; however, when patients lack doctor support, they must take initiative for their own care, as we did.

This is not merely the future of diagnosis – it is the future of medicine.

Given AI's recognised role in medicine, why would a teaching hospital respond judgmentally, condescendingly, and derogatorily when questioned about the potential use of AI to aid in Mikayla's diagnosis?

However, we had everything at stake – so every possibility was open to us.

CHAPTER 14

HOW WE USED AI IN MIKAYLA'S DIAGNOSIS PROCESS

I love innovation—analysing and creating solutions to enable tasks to be performed more effectively. When OpenAI launched ChatGPT in December 2022, I registered within three weeks and began exploring the software to uncover its capabilities. Over the following months and years, the technology improved continuously, and it is exciting to experience its power.

In my business, we had clients who were already using AI for medical diagnostics, making advancements, and contributing to the future of medicine—innovation at its best. So, this concept was not new to me.

In early February, I returned home from another long day at the hospital and collapsed into bed. To calm my mind, I scrolled through my emails. The first one that appeared was a TEDx talk about cardiologists in the US using AI to diagnose complex conditions.

I sat up, jolted into alertness, and became fully engaged in the TEDx talk. It was the most exhilarating fifteen minutes I had experienced in the past eight months. I sensed opportunity, assistance, guidance, relief, and potential. TEDx's slogan is "Ideas change everything." How on point was its marketing team that day! I seized that slogan and dashed to the computer. Another late night at the computer but a complete change in our thinking.

https://www.ted.com/talks/eric_topol_can_ai_catch_what_doctors_miss

Since then, numerous TEDx talks have addressed AI and medical innovations. As discussed in the previous chapter, the true value of AI in medical diagnosis lies in supporting doctors rather than replacing them. However, I turned to AI when the doctors left me with no alternatives. They were unhelpful, and I felt isolated. I needed to support Mikayla. At that moment, it was either me or no one.

Most doctors made light of my use of "googling" and Wikipedia. I realised they misunderstood the difference when they equated AI with Google and Wikipedia. How bold of them to suggest I wasn't aware! There is a clear difference between researching a topic online and brainstorming with AI. This again was the imbalance of power in the patient-doctor relationship re-appearing. Even as something as researching was determined, without asking any questions on what I was researching and where, that I was incapable of understanding the information. Their intent seemed to be for me to question myself, which felt like gaslighting all over again.

I find doctors quite fascinating to analyse. Why would someone choose to gaslight me instead of simply asking a question about my theory or the AI results? Be inquisitive, doctors! Remember, you are not God and do not have all the answers.

I printed copies of all the AI findings for everyone to review. I wanted to encourage the doctors to participate and observe how I directed the conversation. Additionally, I wanted them to acknowledge that the sequence of questions I used was consistent with their usual practice.

Answers arose, as if I had the most knowledgeable medical professionals in the room brainstorming with me, leading to thorough AI responses. We integrated progressive strands of finely tuned results to improve the medical outcomes as supplementary information.

At this stage of Mikayla's medical journey, I had narrowed down the collection of medical journals to over 40 saved copies. There were likely another 50 that were either very close, too outdated, or repeated similar hypotheses. I eliminated those to keep the folder clear. I retained only the relevant material. I printed the essential journals and carried them in the most treasured folder that safeguarded Mikayla's medical documents and information.

Into AI went ... A 19-year-old female presenting with symptoms ... attached were discharge papers, medical journals, and other relevant documents detailing the seizures. Even the spreadsheet has been converted to PDF and uploaded. Now, sit back and wait for approximately 20 seconds. Lean towards the computer; the closer you are to the screen, the quicker the results appear and the more accurate they become!

You need to be specific with your information. In our profession, we have a saying: "Garbage in, garbage out." This is particularly relevant for any AI application.

The first time resulted in six suggestions. Over time, we added more information. Please, AI, consider this request; kindly review it. I'm unsure if the results come back faster when one is polite, but the speed was astounding. I remember thinking we could further expedite this process if I had a doctor beside me. They could utilise their medical knowledge; I needed to consult more medical journals.

Within six weeks, AI had narrowed down the results to two organs as the cause of the seizures. I just needed to find an open-minded doctor. Or should I keep this to myself? I continued, as mentioning "two organs" was somewhat confusing. Where is the connection? I asked AI more questions for clarification, and the intelligent team of virtual medical professionals—my team of medical experts—provided clarity, experience, speed, and an explanation.

It genuinely felt like an anticlimax of emotions. After all this time, it came down to a computer and me. Why do I feel cheated? I should be ecstatic that I figured this out, yet discovering this solution is not my responsibility. I just wanted the doctors to care enough, to see the desperation in my face, to listen to the pain in my voice, and to observe my daughter seizing without stopping. I didn't want to feel clever; I wanted to scream at them.

Ultimately, you need to be brave and confident in the strength of your work. It wasn't challenging for me to tackle a complex problem using a methodical approach.

The outcome was that AI was indeed correct. And guess what – traditional medical diagnostic procedures and tests confirmed this. Did I influence or encourage haste? Yes, let's proceed with that test, fully aware of where it would or should lead.

In a very simplistic explanation, ultimately, one organ was not functioning properly, leading to numerous issues. This impacted organ two then this caused the seizures. A perfect storm one could ask? Or is this a holistic medicine approach – reviewing the body as one machine not as individual pieces.

Although it took another nine months to reach the final diagnosis using the traditional method, we were able to utilise the information for Mikayla, resulting in her experiencing no seizures after March. That was the most significant gift a parent could hope for.

I recognise that there is, and will continue to be, distrust regarding the use of AI for medical diagnosis, for a while to come. We needed to keep the AI knowledge confidential while the medical profession conducted its tests, allowing them to build on the knowledge we had gained.

Constructing this detailed case became almost therapeutic. Documenting each small victory helped me process the overwhelming emotions of fear, anxiety, and exhaustion. It provided a sense of order and a measure of control in a situation that initially felt entirely beyond my grasp. This methodical approach enabled me to channel my grief, anger, and frustration into constructive action – my superpower.

CHAPTER 15

COMPELLING DATA IGNORED

"With hindsight" is a term that usually signifies, well, we messed that up. But does that excuse poor performance or behaviour? One can apply this question to a sports team losing a game they should have won on paper. A common excuse for subpar performance is, "We should have trained harder." In hindsight, the team should have spent more hours in the gym and on the training pitch. That is hindsight.

This analogy can be applied to any situation in which hindsight obscures the valid reason for saying, "We should have trained harder."

Returning to the question: Does hindsight excuse poor performance or behaviour? Ultimately, it is those most affected who shall decide.

Years ago, I had the most remarkable job while recovering from a chronic illness. Executive relocations involved settling international executives in Australia for their employment, usually during the construction of significant projects. We would profile schools, show them houses, attempt to describe Australian culture, explain why there are no kangaroos in the middle of major cities, and mention that spiders are smaller than your shoe.

We addressed any questions related to the new city they were moving to. A lot of driving was involved, and nothing was worse than driving in silence. Fortunately, I possess an inquisitive mind and can converse with nearly anyone.

One day, I met with a safety executive who specialised in mine safety. That same day, a mining accident occurred overseas. Amidst the houses and suburbs, we discussed mine safety for hours. For me, it was a personalised lesson in safety, filled with intriguing concepts and statistics. I should have requested a test to be assessed on the masterclass in safety I had duly attended.

A comment from this expert that has remained with me for over 15 years is that accidents are not genuinely accidental. They can be prevented if someone chooses to act differently or alters the course of an event. If someone takes sufficient care to ask, "Is this right?", they should think carefully about how to proceed with the action.

The notion that altering a trajectory through intervention will prevent or lessen an accident or event is so significant that, theoretically, it could mitigate health repercussions, alter global warming, or halt disease. This principle even extends to family parenting, intervene before a child gets hurt for example. This straightforward concept can avert negative outcomes, including death.

So, why do we hesitate to intervene? Why are we afraid to make change? I expect people to act. If you foresee an outcome likely to harm someone, act, offer guidance, and do something. Stop being a passive observer.

The data was available, yet doctors dismissed it—overlooked it, refused to act on it, ignored it. Whatever the explanation for the outcome, "with hindsight," the medical professionals in the hospital ought to have seen it.

With hindsight, the clues were all in the spreadsheet, the medical journals, the physical consultations, and the information we attempted to convey from family to doctor. However, hindsight is futile, a squandered opportunity, and a waste of life.

There was an occasion in ED, eight months into attendance due to Mikayla's seizures, when we had solid evidence of one of the culprits, and the doctor appeared at the end of the bed in resus. Mikayla was unconscious, so he directed his questions at me.

"What happened today?" was the question. Hence, I began with, "Eight months ago…" almost as if opening a storybook, "Once upon a time." He interrupted me abruptly, saying, "I want to know what happened today."

I felt somewhat taken aback, attempting to explain that there is a backstory and that one must understand the history to appreciate what has brought us here today. "Just tell me what happened today," was the curt reply. In my mind, I thought, "You're a dick," but I don't play poker very well, so I'm sure he got the message.

Taking a deep breath, I say – as you can see, she's having seizures. I telepathically urge Mikayla to wake up; I must get you out of here. Where's that wheelbarrow?

In hindsight, it didn't matter how much compelling data I had collected; it was all about attitude: the attitude to recognise that others can contribute to a solution, the attitude to appreciate the value that all team members bring to the war room, and the attitude and belief that everyone adds some level of value to solving problems. Some minor pieces of the puzzle ultimately create the whole jigsaw.

The sheer volume of data meticulously compiled in my ever-growing folder was wasted on those who lacked the mindset to believe that anyone without a medical degree could contribute. Listening is an incredibly undervalued skill; one learns so much when one listens and asks questions.

At one point, I successfully persuaded a neurologist to review a test result. She returned the following day, confidently asserting that her FND diagnosis was accurate and that it was unrelated to blood sugar. In hindsight, she was mistaken.

What did not happen was that she didn't review the spreadsheet, didn't take the time to understand the pre-seizure activities and the lack of food, and didn't discuss my findings with me. Moreover, she focused exclusively on one set of figures as isolated results, rather than viewing them within a broader context.

What she also didn't acknowledge is that when the body seizes, there is a stress release that can increase blood sugar levels. So, when she was reading levels 3, which is still below the minimum of 4, there was no consideration of the stress response to the body. But why did I need to find that out? It was all about attitude.

She could have gazed at the beautiful graphs, yearning to be removed from the folder. They longed to break free and share their tale. I suspect she merely went through the motions to keep me quiet.

Perhaps the most damning piece of evidence was the sheer frequency and severity of the seizures. Two hundred seizures in a relatively short period are not the typical presentation. This was not merely a matter of minor variations; this was an outlier, a data point so far removed from the norm that it raised serious questions about the diagnosis.

Despite the overwhelming weight of contrary evidence, the persistence of the FND diagnosis was deeply troubling. It felt as if our reality and lived experience were being actively ignored, dismissed as the anxieties of an overwrought parent.

The emotional toll of this relentless dismissal was immeasurable. Exhaustion, frustration, and fear intertwined in a suffocating web of stress that threatened to engulf us. We were left feeling unheard and invisible; our voices lost to an indifferent machine of the healthcare system.

What made the experience even more disheartening was the palpable sense of gaslighting that permeated interactions with numerous medical professionals. It felt as though our observations and concerns were being actively minimised, dismissed as mere parental anxieties, or, even worse, as evidence of some inherent flaw in our judgement or character. This dismissal went beyond simple disagreement; it represented a systematic, insidious attempt to undermine our narrative and reinforce their initial diagnosis, irrespective of the mounting evidence.

CHAPTER 16

DIFFICULT CONVERSATIONS WITH DOCTORS

It was a rookie mistake. I had confidence that the doctors and I were part of Mikayla's team, and my steadfast belief of this remained unshakeable for at least three months.

In my world, my team and I operate across 30 industries and interact with hundreds of diverse personalities. Did you know that individuals in specific industry positions often exhibit similar personality traits? We know how to draw out the highest performance from various personality types to achieve the best project outcomes. Isolating subject matter experts typically results in poor outcomes in projects with tight deadlines, which is not ideal.

I have collaborated with doctors, professors, researchers, and exceptionally talented individuals in their respective fields for many years. However, I was there to fulfil a role in which they recognised my capabilities and expertise in comparison to their own. We worked as a team to achieve a shared goal, which ensured our communication was founded on mutual and equal respect. More importantly, it was a reciprocal process, leading to successful projects.

Introduce the doctor-patient relationship. This feels like a wet fish slap across the face.

In my ignorance, I assumed that doctors possessed superior communication skills when interacting with patients. The ability to extract clues is crucial; let's be honest: ask 100 people to describe something, and you will receive 100 different explanations. The explanation is subjective.

This is particularly pertinent for emergency doctors, as they have access to a patient's medical history. Different countries have diverse laws governing patient medical information. Nevertheless, the initial course of investigation remains the same: collect as many clues as possible that are relevant to the presenting illness.

But what happens if the patient records contain a documented diagnosis? Does this affect an individual's opinion? Human nature suggests that it does. What if that opinion comes from a colleague in your field? What happens if you have doubts, yet the "system" does not support them or permit you to challenge the prevailing view or express an opinion?

The result will be conflict.

My greatest challenge was convincing the doctors that the information I was trying to share with them was valuable. First, as they continually reminded me—and rightly so—I was not a doctor. Second, they firmly adhered to the FND diagnosis provided by their colleagues, even without questioning that initial diagnosis. They had no reason to listen to the mother; the doctors abundantly clarified that.

Communication can be verbal—referring to the words used—or nonverbal, encompassing actions and body language. The doctors utilised both aspects through their tone of voice, choice of words, and physical behaviours, such as rolling their eyes or appearing unresponsive. Their communication made their opinion obvious.

One night, in the resuscitation bed, the ED doctor stood with his arms crossed and said, "There is nothing we can do for an FND diagnosis." "But it isn't FND," I replied, "you are doing nothing!" Then came seizure nine. That night, Mikayla was transferred to the high-dependency unit in the ICU because she kept seizing repeatedly.

On the walk to the ward, he behaved like a spoiled child who had lost a card game. He didn't speak to me, his arms crossed. In contrast, when I'm stressed, I use laughter as a coping mechanism. Thus, the more his body language communicated clear messages about how unhappy he was about transporting a patient for whom he believed nothing could be done, the more I responded with humour.

Nothing was amusing about that night; my only other emotion was tears. However, I couldn't shed tears, as I would then be labelled an emotional and potentially irrational mother. Moreover, no one takes emotional people seriously.

Aside from the initial visit to the emergency department, only one doctor demonstrated genuine interest in listening and engaging in two-way communication. He allowed me to clearly explain the symptoms detailed in the spreadsheet. However, a system that does not permit deviation or discussion hindered him. Mikayla remained unconscious the entire time from when she was transferred by the ambulance paramedics directly into another resuscitation bed.

Then there was the remarkable nurse who, one night, once again by a resuscitation bed, quietly approached and stood beside me. She whispered, 'You are onto something; do not give up; keep going.'

It was the most explicit message, something she was probably not allowed to say. Yet here was someone brave enough to express encouragement, someone I cherish, who had the courage to share those words, someone who ventured beyond the confines of the establishment.

The bullying was so severe that I taught Mikayla strategies to counter physical communication while I managed the verbal aspects.

One neurologist excelled in physical communication; he would sit at the end of the bed, speak to Mikayla in simple English, and provide clear explanations. Although he explained the FND diagnosis, he truly showcased his communication strengths. I coached her to ensure she sat up straight in bed, attempted to position herself as close to eye level as possible, and elevated the bed. When feasible, she should project her voice powerfully and pose direct questions.

A common question that health professionals often ask is, "How are you today?" For anyone not confined to a hospital bed, the answer can be vague and is typically, "Great, how are you?" This response signifies no commitment and offers no insight into one's true feelings. How does one respond when they are unwell and trying to maintain a positive mindset? The outcome is usually not accurate.

But how does one communicate when one party is fixated on a single solution, while the other insists they haven't questioned it sufficiently? Conflict arises. Such conflict was present at every point of contact. It didn't matter how many medical journals or A4 sheets the spreadsheet contained; when one party refuses to listen, discuss, and consider another option, all is lost.

Ryan's Rule in Queensland and Martha's Rule in the UK—both laws born from the tragic deaths of children due to doctors' inaction. These cases involve coroners assessing avoidable fatalities. I can see Mikayla deteriorating, so I called the number. I dialled that number three times that night, and two hours later, someone appeared at her bedside. So much for the promised 30-minute response time.

They didn't bother to ask about my concerns; instead, they informed me that he had reviewed her file and was following protocol. He wasn't a doctor; they sent a nurse as the messenger. There were no questions, no communication—a scripted and prepared response. What am I facing? Please get me that wheelbarrow.

This experience became the norm. Each conversation felt like scaling an insurmountable wall. We presented our data, observations, and fears, only to be met with polite yet firm rejections. Some doctors were dismissive, while others condescended. A few showed genuine empathy, yet their attempts to assist were often undermined by the prevailing consensus supporting the initial diagnosis. We were running in circles, the medical carousel spinning endlessly, providing no respite from the ongoing seizures.

The frustration became unbearable, eroding our emotional resilience. We were being gaslighted, subtly yet effectively; our experiences minimised, and our concerns dismissed as mere anxiety.

We learned to anticipate dismissive responses and prepare counterarguments supported by facts and figures. We also learned to be assertive without being aggressive and to advocate without being perceived as overly complex. We didn't want security to be called in.

I cannot overstate the emotional toll of these confrontations. The weight of responsibility, the fear for Mikayla's safety, and the financial burden create an atmosphere of constant stress and anxiety. Sleepless nights became the norm, punctuated by the jarring sounds of seizures that shook our home and our hearts. What was that thumping noise? Is Mikayla on the floor? "Mikayla – are you OK?" was the constant cry, as I held my breath until she answered.

We realised our persistent advocacy was about obtaining an accurate diagnosis and ensuring that other families would not endure the same challenges and suffering.

Our family unit grew stronger, and our bonds were forged in the crucible of shared adversity. We stood together, united against a formidable foe, our love fuelling our unwavering commitment to justice. The fight was far from over, but we knew, with absolute certainty, that we would continue to fight until we achieved a just outcome.

PART FOUR

CHAPTER 17

THE WILD AND WONDERFUL COMMENTS

These individual comments from specialists, doctors, nurses, and hospital management often go unnoticed when viewed in isolation, as single one-off comments or as a single time in hospital. However, for Mikayla and our family, they were a constant presence. Some expressed their views in a single sentence, others retorted when they felt too many questions were being asked, and some were extraordinarily unprofessional. Three could have resulted in her death if we had listened. Some, and repeatedly said, were potentially in breach of the Australian Charter of Healthcare Rights.

At times, our confusion led to utter silence. Some comments were made deliberately and strategically to create divisions within the family. Here are the most memorable examples. Many of these remarks were spoken in front of several family members, so they are not merely seen as "misunderstandings." They are neither taken out of context nor misheard or misinterpreted. There were other remarks—these are simply the most notable interactions.

1. You just need to accept FND – multiple neurologists multiple times.
2. You do not need to call an ambulance – multiple neurologists multiple times.
3. There is no need to come to hospital – there is nothing we can do – multiple neurologists multiple times.
4. You should stay at home – multiple neurologists.
5. I have known this Dr, and if she says it is FND, then I trust her; there is nothing I can do – cardiologist 18 hours after a consult and then speaking to the neurologist.
6. How many boyfriends does your Mum bring home? – neurologist.
7. Your Mum must be so busy and ignores you – neurologist.
8. It is not blood-sugar-related – neurologist.
9. It is not our responsibility to see how much she eats – neurology nurse.
10. We only do the normal blood tests – ED doctor.
11. We don't test for other blood results – ED doctor.
12. She is not sick enough to be admitted – ED doctor.
13. He is doing a fishing expedition – neurologist regarding tests requested by another doctor in the private sector.
14. She will grow out of it – ED doctors.
15. My daughter went 18 months fainting – ED doctor.
16. What do you want me to do? – ED doctors?
17. There is nothing we can do – ED doctors.
18. Don't let her seize on the ground; it is dirty – ED nurse.
19. We don't have funding to admit her – gastroenterologist regarding who should admit – endocrinology or gastroenterology.
20. It is Mikayla's illness – she is to answer – nurse unit manager, neurologists, and ED doctors (often demanded when Mikayla had just regained consciousness and was only able to nod her head)

21. She is not unconscious, just not responsive – ED doctors; neurologists after 22 hours unconscious, downplaying the actuality.
22. It is FND – a neurologist from a different hospital after being advised that if you want her to seize, encourage her to run around the ward and use energy.
23. Quoted phrases that are the recommended statements from the FND Learning Guide for Nurses – multiple nurses and multiple doctors.

    a. I see a lot of patients with similar problems – heading in the document "Suggested for use when explaining what they have".
    b. Imagine the hardware of a computer is intact, but there is a software problem – heading in document "Metaphors and comparisons can be helpful".
    c. Something like a short circuit in your nervous system – another metaphor from the training guide.
    d. I do not think you are imagining or putting on the symptoms – heading of "Indicate that you believe them".
    e. I see a lot of patients with a similar problem – heading of "Emphasise that it is common".

Hospital staff often referred to other sayings from the playbook. We were unaware that the training book existed and were puzzled when the staff were using the exact phrases verbatim. It felt odd that they were all saying the same things. One night, while researching, I stumbled upon it by chance. It was the resource they were using to lead my daughter to question, pressure her into accepting an inaccurate diagnosis, and doubt herself—to gaslight her.

CHAPTER 18

PATIENT ADVOCACY

The exhaustion was bone deep. Twenty-one visits to the emergency room. Thirty specialists. Two hundred seizures. The relentless cycle had worn us down, leaving us emotionally and financially drained. We had faced dismissal, doubt, and the insidious erosion of hope.

Patient advocacy should bridge the gap between the medical establishment and individuals, such as Mikayla and our family. It should hold the system accountable and empower people to navigate the complexities of healthcare.

Patient advocacy goes beyond simply supporting a condition-specific cause. While organisations dedicated to illnesses concentrate on research, treatments, and community support, patient advocacy seeks systemic change. It ensures that all patients receive timely, respectful, and effective care, regardless of their diagnosis. It is vital to recognise the existence of these organisations.

It had been ten months without anyone informing us about patient advocacy management in the hospital. However, that position was not established to help advocate for patients – quite the opposite. It was a role designed to defend the hospital's actions as being entirely responsible. In fact – no, you haven't any patient advocacy in the hospital, either of them we went to.

Advocacy shouldn't be this draining. When standard protocols fail, systems should protect patients. Formal advocacy frameworks like Ryan's Rule (QLD), Martha's Rule (UK), REACH (NSW), Aishwarya's CARE Call (WA) are essential.

These laws are not established if the system had functioned to support patients. But there are. In Australia, and in the United Kingdom. Laws won't change the fundamental systemic problems that caused these awful and avoidable deaths. The problem is partly attitudinal.

Ryan's Rule was implemented in Queensland, Australia, following the tragic death of Ryan Saunders, a young boy who lost his life to an undiagnosed and untreated streptococcal infection, despite his family's persistent efforts to obtain prompt medical care. Ryan's Rule enables patients and their families to express concerns if they believe their condition is deteriorating and their issues are not being addressed. A patient or caregiver can initiate an independent clinical review by calling a specific number, prompting the medical team to reassess the situation to ensure that no critical issues are overlooked.

A similar mechanism would have been advantageous for us. Countless times, we witnessed doctors overlooking clear signs of deterioration, resulting in our return to the emergency department just days later. Implementing a structured escalation process could have spared us numerous nights filled with fear, anxiety, and frustration.

Martha's Rule, inspired by Ryan's Rule, was proposed in the UK following the tragic passing of 13-year-old Martha Mills, whose sepsis was overlooked despite clear warning signs. Her parents expressed concerns about her deteriorating health, but these were ignored by medical staff. The proposed rule ensures that patients and their families have the legal right to seek an urgent second opinion from a different medical team if they feel their concerns are not being addressed or heard.

These laws reflected our own in disturbing ways—the agonising awareness of an issue yet feeling helpless due to medical apathy. Implementing a formal rule enabling families to seek an independent review could avert numerous tragedies and uphold the notion that no parent should have to fight to be heard or taken seriously.

New South Wales has launched a similar initiative called REACH (Recognise, Engage, Act, Call, Help). This programme allows patients and their families to express concerns when they feel their health issues are not being managed appropriately. It outlines a clear intervention procedure, enabling swift reassessment and prioritisation of urgent cases.

This system is established, yet it still failed us. A system's strength relies heavily on human execution. I could go on about dismissiveness, condescension, and numerous other negative behaviours, but if someone had taken our REACH calls seriously, then 200 seizures would have been a lot fewer. Advocacy shouldn't fall only on desperate parents; the system must recognise it as a core part of patient care.

Advocacy should encompass organised referral systems, improved transparency in medical records, and AI-supported diagnostics to eliminate human bias from the process. Advocacy could have aided in obtaining:

MEDICAL RECORD ACCESSIBILITY

Patients should have unrestricted access to their medical histories in real time to avoid omissions and distortions that may occur during referral letters.

Advocacy could have assisted in believing that AI could help.

AI-ASSISTED DIAGNOSTICS

AI technology should be integrated with medical professionals to analyse patient data and identify patterns that might be overlooked. This could significantly reduce misdiagnoses and expedite appropriate treatment care.

Mikayla's health struggle uncovered significant flaws in the system that require attention. Patient advocacy means voicing concerns for those in distress, seeking responsibility, and ensuring that families aren't forced to manage a malfunctioning system alone.

By establishing formal escalation processes, enhancing patient advocacy networks with advocates there for the family, and adopting technological innovations, we can foster a future where advocacy transforms from a desperate challenge into a fundamental, unquestioned right for everyone.

No one should have to endure the same struggle we faced merely to be heard, only to remain unheard.

CHAPTER 19

COMPLAINTS AND FORMAL GRIEVANCES

My frustration surpasses all my previous experiences. Typically, I excel at managing conflict and guiding others through challenges. However, I continuously encountered a communication barrier when interacting with doctors, nurses, hospital management, government officials, and health complaint organisations. They outright rejected meaningful dialogue. Even during conversations, they spoke at me, dismissing my responses.

At one stage, we encountered a significant issue with a neurologist, prompting me to arrange a meeting with the NUM and other staff, about six people in the meeting. Mikayla's father travelled from interstate urgently when Mikayla was in ICU and unconscious for 22 hours, so he was available to attend this meeting as well. After an hour of discussion, they reached several agreements—most crucially, that one particular neurologist would have no further contact with Mikayla.

We left the meeting feeling assured that they would honour their commitment. Yet, that afternoon, who should enter the room? That neurologist! I was infuriated—such a waste of time and energy, and why did we bother trying to work as a team. It quickly became apparent that the meeting was merely a "smokescreen" pretending to address concerns, alter behaviours, and propose modifications. However, there was no genuine intention to enact any change.

When I perceive something as unfair or unfulfilled, my immediate reaction isn't to complain or engage in discussion. Addressing a concern is not the same as complaining; don't whinge about it if you aren't prepared to express the issue.

When I raise an issue, I try to offer several mutually beneficial solutions to tackle it. Solving problems is my greatest strength—my true superpower. Merely complaining isn't effective because it depends on the other person being as committed to helping you as you are to pointing out the issue.

Being in the neurology ward was shocking; most patients had suffered strokes. It was more often referred as the stroke ward. The patient mix was predominately elderly, and there was a mix of genders. As we entered the ward, I could sense the horror of what lay ahead. That was another reason I stayed at the hospital every day for as long as I could – to ensure Mikayla wasn't affected by what she was witnessing. However, it was a public hospital; she was there for a reason, so we bunkered down and endured.

Until she was placed in a ward with three men over seventy-five, each at varying stages of cognitive ability, the curtains were drawn to ensure maximum privacy. However, the hospital staff opened the curtain upon entering, revealing a man older than Mikayla's grandfather, his gown undone and everything on display.

I gasped, tossed the laptop onto the bed, and jumped out of the chair to close the curtain. Turning to Mikayla, I noticed her silently mouthing words to me. My thoughts raced—surely this isn't allowed;

there must be rules for mixed wards. She was only 19, for goodness' sake.

Naturally, there should be a procedure. I understood that although it was a hospital, it was still an organisation, and all organisations have procedures. My approach involves gathering information to devise a solution; otherwise, I'm simply complaining.

Of course, publicly available, there is a State specific procedure concerning mixed genders in wards and the responsibilities of nursing staff. It is not a mandatory procedure, unlike how to avoid killing or maiming someone. Nevertheless, it remains a procedure that employees or contractors commit to following in their employment or engagement agreements. That is normal in all organisations and businesses – for staff and contractors to accept the company rules – their policies and procedures.

I approached the desk the following day and asked to speak to the person in charge. I calmly outlined the issue and asked if she could assist in finding a solution. Her response was clear: No, we are at capacity. The initial step was to recognise her reply and offer an alternative solution.

The other solution is when "the next bed is available." This ward comprises 32 beds, approximately six single rooms, with the remainder configured as four-bed arrangements. This was a busy ward with high patient volume, and patient turnover was constant: in, out, in, out. We spent considerable time in that ward, learning its operations. We had hundreds of hours to observe a great deal – and we observed a lot.

She refused to help, so I always saved the trump card until the end. The procedure then emerged. I mentioned the procedure's name and emphasised the section that clarified what they needed to do.

I didn't have to slide my finger along the page to point out the bright yellow highlights. Her response was, "We will see what we can do." That translates to inaction, and as anticipated, nothing occurred.

Just imagine your 19-year-old daughter being exposed to the genitalia of 75+-year-old men or not wearing shirts or with their gowns wide open.

Nonetheless, there were times when raising an issue led to formal complaints. We filed a complaint with the Health Care Complaints Commission (HCCC), which addresses health complaints in New South Wales. Similar organisations exist in every state and relevant country. I am confident in my writing ability—the complaints were clear and concise, and I express myself even under pressure.

It seemed like an act of rebellion. How terrible must I be for voicing my concerns about the health system, which I had always trusted not to fail me publicly and privately? However, this experience was unprecedented, and I am profoundly disheartened by what the hospital and health system have become.

I voiced my concerns several times, but it became absurd, so I ultimately gave up due to their lack of assistance. When I finally received a response, it was merely a standard letter, a generic acknowledgement of my complaint without genuine engagement with its content.

The dismissal was subtle yet tangible, reflecting a bureaucratic indifference that deepened our frustration and helplessness. This was far from the meaningful engagement, genuine concern, or proactive investigation we had anticipated. It felt like yet another obstacle, yet another challenge in our already arduous journey.

Hospitals employ patient advocates, but from our experience they primarily serve the hospital's interests rather than those of the patients, often prioritising silence over support for the individuals seeking care.

I contacted the Premier, the Health Minister, local MPs, and lawyers but received no response. I later learned from their reply email that I had contacted the wrong MP electorate.

These experiences compelled me to seek Mikayla's diagnosis on my own. I felt utterly alone as I navigated the vast hospital with no one to assist me. Despite the available resources, I found myself without support, and if anything, they seemed to hinder rather than help.

CHAPTER 20

EXPLORING OPTIONS FOR ACCOUNTABILITY

Accountability signifies responsibility, yet many individuals often evade it. This trend extends beyond the medical and health fields, impacting businesses and organisations worldwide. Accountability inherently involves vulnerability—how can one confess to errors without recognising their weaknesses? As a result, people frequently avoid accountability unless forced to confront it.

Accountability assumes various forms and yields different outcomes depending on the circumstances.

Our leaders fail to instil accountability through their actions. One could spend days citing examples of leaders evading true responsibility, this is a global issue not just Australia. Voters, shareholders, and employees have become accustomed to their excuses, but that should not be an excuse for leaders to evade facing the truth. They hide away because they dislike being held responsible.

We expect everyone to be perfect, so we create systems, procedures, reporting lines, and corporate structures to ensure that individuals are accountable to each other. However, is this proper accountability or just a form of it?

This raises the question of whether taking responsibility is assumed when a mistake occurs.

Underneath accountability, a troubling truth emerges – Gaslighting, the manipulation and aggression faced by patients. These actions act as a cancer within the healthcare system, where the stakes involve life and death.

Patients questioning their diagnoses, voicing concerns, or requesting second opinions frequently encounter dismissal, invalidation, or outright hostility. Gaslighting is a tactic that causes patients to doubt their symptoms or experiences, eroding trust in the healthcare system and discouraging them from taking charge of their health. Bullying, which can manifest as condescension, coercion, or intimidation, creates a setting in which patients feel disempowered instead of empowered.

Proper accountability in healthcare cannot flourish in an environment where patients feel disregarded or silenced when they seek clarification and support. Tackling these fundamental issues is equally important as implementing accountability measures and structures. Organisations and leaders must alter their approach to accountability to foster positive change rather than instil fear. They must:

Foster a culture of psychological safety where patients feel comfortable expressing concerns and asking questions without fear of retaliation.

- Encourage open discussions where healthcare professionals recognise mistakes and uncertainties while prioritising transparency and trust.
- Distinguish between accountability and blame to ensure the medical profession is held accountable, prioritising learning and

improvement over the assignment of fault and guilt.
- Address toxic practices to eliminate the gaslighting and bullying of patients, which is essential for true accountability.

How does the medical profession confront centuries of belief in its infallibility? This perception, which regards the medical field as almost divine, often overlooks the fact that society has evolved beyond accepting subpar and dismissive diagnoses; people now recognise that something deeper is at play.

As I have repeatedly informed the doctors throughout our journey: "You are not God; stop pretending that you are." Oh, and please note, "Mother disagrees with the diagnosis." in Mikayla's patient records.

KAREN PERKS

CHAPTER 21

BULLYING AND GASLIGHTING

The deceptive nature of gaslighting revealed itself disturbingly as we navigated through the medical system. It was not one overt act of deceit, but rather a gradual, intentional undermining of our perception of reality. It began subtly, with dismissive remarks cloaked in medical terminology. "That's typical," one neurologist remarked, brushing aside my growing concerns about the increasingly frequent seizures.

Another dismissed my comprehensive notes on the seizure activity as "anecdotal." A distinct pattern emerged: our observations were minimised, our concerns were labelled as overreactions, and our urgent requests for a more thorough investigation for the physical causes of the seizures faced polite yet firm resistance.

The gaslighting was not always explicit. Often, it involved a subtle shift in dialogue, cleverly diverting attention from our primary concerns. When we presented a new symptom, a behavioural change, or any alarming issue, the doctor would pivot to an unrelated topic. This persistent redirection—this skilful evasion of the actual problem—

constituted a form of gaslighting, deftly employed to prevent us from questioning the initial diagnosis.

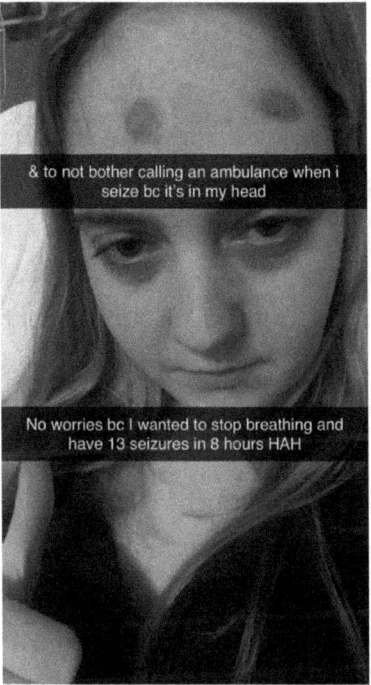

Mikayla knew there was gaslighting.

The cumulative effects of these interactions proved devastating. Doubt seeped into our perceptions. The confidence that once stemmed from parental instincts—that steadfast belief in our understanding of Mikayla—began to diminish under constant dismissals. The relentless scrutiny of our observations and the insidious undermining of our experiences gradually eroded our self-esteem and diminished our capacity to advocate for Mikayla's well-being.

We second-guessed our feelings, wondering if we were overreacting, overly dramatic, or imagining things. The ongoing necessity of justifying our concerns and validating our observations added a tiring burden of emotional labour to an already unbearable situation.

However we had our records, the spreadsheet to remind us we were not overreacting. Not being an overly emotional parent, not being difficult.

Gaslighting infiltrated various aspects of our lives, extending beyond direct encounters with healthcare providers. Acknowledging gaslighting was our initial step in combating it. It prompted us to continue to meticulously record everything: the seizure dates and times, descriptions of episodes, medical professionals' responses, and any other pertinent details. This record became essential in our advocacy, providing objective evidence physicians could not easily dismiss or overlook.

Additionally, we discovered how to express our concerns more assertively. Rather than simply reporting observations, we actively questioned diagnoses and treatment plans. We learned to pose direct enquiries, challenge medical professionals, and insist they support their conclusions with specific evidence, promoting a more thorough approach to diagnosis and treatment.

We recognised that our often-overlooked parental intuition was a crucial and valuable part of Mikayla's healthcare. Our persistent questions, bolstered by documented evidence, became effective for addressing subtle and overt gaslighting manipulations.

The journey proved challenging and emotionally draining. At times, we felt defeated and overwhelmed by the situation's burden, which led us to doubt our ability to persevere. Despite being a long and complex battle, the experience provided crucial insights into the intricacies of the medical system and underscored the importance of proactive patient advocacy.

Our narrative serves as a rallying cry, urging fellow parents and patients to recognise the deceptive tactics of gaslighting and to assert their rights within the healthcare system with bravery.

CHAPTER 22

STRATEGIES FOR SELF-PRESERVATION

I have always believed that when faced with an obstacle, confronting it directly isn't always necessary; instead, one can find a way around it. This was my approach while navigating the emergency department and proceeding to neurology. I realised that some doctors, nurses, management, and patient advocate executives were not my allies in Mikayla's journey; they were hurdles—daunting, exhausting, sometimes insurmountable, but mainly just barriers blocking the path. No matter how many tactics I employed, I couldn't shift them. So, I chose to leave them behind and chart my own course. This became the foundation for my self-preservation strategy.

They continually undermined our confidence, but I found ways to restore it and remain focused. This typically happened after my sessions in what I referred to as the "intervention lounge." I occasionally doubted myself, questioning whether I was overreacting. However, each time I witnessed her suffer another seizure, I recognised with complete certainty that I was not.

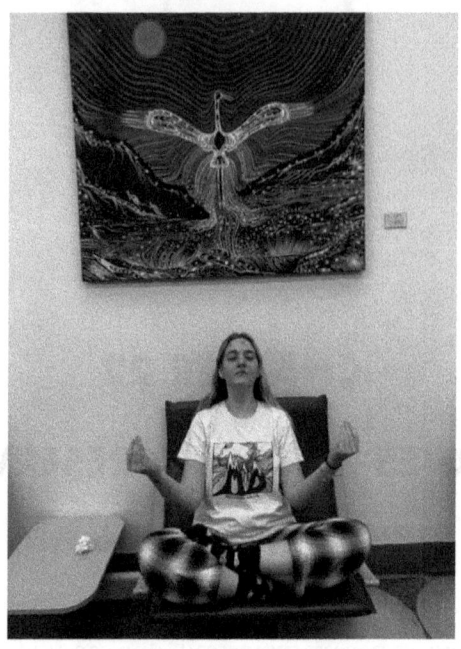

Mikayla doing mindfulness in the hospital. We coped with humour.

The spreadsheet served as my armour against gaslighting. More than just documentation, it became a weapon, a shield, and a lifeline. It preserved the truth when others refuted it, standing firm as undeniable evidence against the condescending attitudes we encountered. It recorded everything—triggers, patterns, medical visits, and indisputable proof that Mikayla's condition was genuine. When another doctor attempted to disregard us, I could present solid data—pages detailing 200 seizures and numerous medical appointments. They couldn't contest that. They couldn't overlook what was directly in front of them.

I had to adjust my speaking style, as I had previously employed more submissive language. Being assertive didn't equate to being aggressive; it focused on clear communication. I stripped emotion from my words, not because I wasn't experiencing it but to prevent medical professionals from using my feelings against me. I practised my responses, anticipated objections, and constructed my arguments as a lawyer would prepare for a case. I transformed into a presence that could not be overlooked or intimidated.

Throughout this journey, I had to prioritise my well-being; the emotional burden of feeling dismissed, doubted, and overlooked while witnessing my child's suffering was overwhelming. Therapy became my sanctuary for unravelling the gaslighting, recognising it for what it truly was, and restoring the parts of myself that had been diminished. Therapy helped me realise that my doubt wasn't genuinely my own; instead, it was instilled by a system that sought to make me question myself. It restored my confidence, sanity, and a deeper sense of empowerment and self-worth.

Then came self-care, which I initially viewed as a luxury but later realised was essential for survival. If I reached burnout, I wouldn't be able to support Mikayla, Alana, or Reece. Therefore, I dedicated small moments to breathing. A book, a walk, a quiet pause—these were not merely indulgences; they were lifelines. The struggle was prolonged, and I needed to persevere.

Establishing boundaries became the crucial final step. I learned to recognise and address the signs of gaslighting before they took hold. I ceased engaging in discussions that challenged our reality. Whenever someone attempted to downplay our concerns, I interrupted—assertively and without apology. I would no longer go along with it, and no more time would be wasted. I had a purpose and was determined not to allow anyone to divert me from it.

Standing up to gaslighting is a struggle for your mental health, self-confidence, and the welfare of those you care about. It's draining, ongoing, and often maddening. Yet, we have made the system pay attention by documenting our experiences, remaining persistent, communicating assertively, seeking community support, prioritising self-care, and establishing clear boundaries. We found the answers. We secured the treatment. We triumphed.

The scars from this battle will forever linger, but they symbolise more than just pain—they demonstrate our resilience. Our experience uncovered the weaknesses in a system designed to safeguard us. Instead, it compelled us to advocate for what should have been provided without struggle. At the very least, our narrative serves as both a cautionary tale and an inspiration to other, potentially hope—a roadmap for other families traversing the same daunting path. Ultimately, we didn't merely endure; we prevailed.

PART FIVE

CHAPTER 23

AN ACCURATE DIAGNOSIS FINALLY REVEALED

I was not aware of FND when the doctors assigned it to Mikayla during her first hospital stay. Initially, while examining the flow diagram about seizures that had been given to me, I reacted strongly with a "no" when the doctor mentioned the psychological triggers associated with FND. It wasn't that it was a physiological illness, it was because the brochure very clearly stated that seizures can be caused by physical or psychological triggers.

Six months later, I also considered the explanation indicating a fear of vomiting as a stress trigger. Finally, I consulted other psychologists who explained that FND is not typically the first diagnosis made before excluding other physical causes.

The primary challenge I faced with doctors during Mikayla's illness was their lack of interest in investigating the physical causes of her seizures. Instead, they quickly shifted their attention to mental health and psychological factors. Once they recorded FND in her medical files, she was unjustly labelled, which exacerbated the issue.

Is mental health automatically seen as the diagnosis when individuals struggle to face challenging health conditions? The purpose of my initial research was to understand what FND involved. Vague descriptions from doctors only deepened my conviction that they genuinely did not grasp the issue. The explanations that characterised FND as a catch-all for conditions without apparent physical cause left me perplexed. Just because you don't know what the issue is, don't use FND as a default diagnosis.

I began my research within the NHS (UK) system. When Mikayla received the label, the NHS brochure had been confidently presented. That was the first warning sign: Why are we issuing a UK document in an Australian hospital?

What are the statistics on FND diagnoses? Is this diagnosis currently seen as a trend? And why is the hospital that diagnosed Mikayla treating it as if it is "just another one"? Is it just another one?

When I mentioned Mikayla's other physical symptoms—nausea from eating, low iron levels, and fatigue—doctors dismissed me. They ignored my input and treated my family as if we were obstructing their medical expertise. However, her iron levels were so dangerously low that an iron infusion was administered during a hospital stay.

Following the instructions in the UK brochure, I adhered closely to the diagram. My research revealed that, despite Mikayla's FND diagnosis, she was not receiving the care recommended by FND organisations and specialists. No multidisciplinary approach or management plan was implemented; only mindfulness and exercise were advised. More of a general – if you would like to approach.

We were also advised against calling an ambulance due to a perceived lack of necessity and told to avoid the hospital, as it would serve no real purpose. "It won't help," they insisted. "Just stay home and wait it out." I was shocked to learn that having someone unconscious for 22 hours and having seizures was considered acceptable. It felt as though the avenues for help were closing off around us. However, this instruction was never included in the FND brochures, and with very good reason.

We discovered that the most effective way to manage FND is through a collaborative approach involving neurologists, physiotherapists, psychologists, and occupational therapists. However, we had only one solitary GP who was understanding. He acknowledged that he felt overwhelmed by the situation. We were navigating this alone and without guidance.

We endeavoured to embrace FND but found it difficult to grasp its reasoning. How can one accept something without understanding? The era when patients followed doctors' advice without question is over. In the 21st century, we possess technology, reliable information from government sources, Google, and artificial intelligence (AI). These resources enable individuals to access medical journals and health-related information.

These sources should not be regarded as substitutes for medical professionals; however, they certainly provide reliable information in the intricate realm of medical knowledge. Consequently, despite our sincere attempts to understand and potentially accept FND, the diagnosis still left us feeling uneasy and uncertain about its validity.

One ordinary afternoon, we sat together with steaming mugs of tea in hand, discussing everything except the medical turmoil in our lives. Or so we believed.

Unbeknownst to us, the puzzle pieces started to align in our minds. The triggers, patterns, and symptoms that didn't correspond with FND were all mingling in our thoughts, awaiting their resolution.

Suddenly, it emerged. We began to detail everything – the symptoms and, crucially, the relationship between exercise and the seizures, the discrepancies in the diagnosis, and the lack of improvement despite adhering to the recommendations. It became evident that we had identified a pattern, prompting us to organise our findings in a spreadsheet rather than a diary, enabling a concise summary. This spreadsheet allowed us to convert the patterns into graphs, facilitating quick access to information if anyone takes the time to review them. I even employed colour coding for better visual clarity, yet no one showed interest in examining those unfortunate outcomes.

With the help of AI, an Internal Specialist that listened, eventually, the accurate diagnosis unveiled two medical conditions that clarified everything: the symptoms, the triggers, and the lack of response to treatment. It wasn't FND—it was something entirely different, something that could be treated.

Yet, the path to that moment was beginning; we still faced challenges in the public hospital until the private medical system could align. We alternated between the public system each time she experienced clusters of seizures, knowing they were inflexible about their FND diagnosis, and the private system to navigate the complexities of diagnosing.

After a family member's recommendation, we consulted the first internal physician based on our GP's referral. Our symptoms had become increasingly unmanageable, and our frustration with the FND diagnosis had reached its peak. Known for his thoroughness and empathy, we held high hopes that he could provide some clarity. From the moment we entered his office, it was evident that he was dedicated to seeking comprehensive answers rather than simply accepting the easiest ones.

His first evaluation was thorough and unhurried. During a three-hour appointment, he meticulously reviewed every detail of Mikayla's medical history, posed insightful questions, and listened attentively to our concerns, instilling a sense of hope. He concluded that "This is not FND" but emphasised the necessity of acting like detectives to uncover the underlying cause.

"He's very thorough," we remarked, feeling relieved. However, there was a downside to having our highly sought-after internal specialist. His expertise made it difficult to secure follow-up appointments, and in the meantime, conditions continued to worsen. Symptoms grew increasingly unmanageable, and life felt as though it was spiralling out of control. This doctor proposed a potential lead – a likely gastrointestinal issue – and recommended both an endoscopy and a colonoscopy to rule out or confirm any gastrointestinal abnormalities that could be driving this cascade of symptoms.

Preparing for the procedures required fasting, which was a challenge we hadn't anticipated. I had already begun to theorise that energy use equates to seizures. However, it wasn't until recovery that we realised how crucial this insight would prove to be.

Following the procedures during recovery, the unimaginable occurred –not just one seizure, but multiple episodes. They were severe enough to require an urgent transfer to the ICU at the nearby private hospital. This distressing experience prompted further investigations and consultations with our secondary internal specialist. Fortunately, Mikayla remained safe that night, allowing me to return home for some rest.

The first meeting with him was surprising. His relaxed demeanour and keen intellect offered comfort, and during our initial discussion, we realised he was genuinely listening.

We continued to meticulously record all data in a spreadsheet, including meals, activity levels, symptoms, and the frequency and severity of seizures. The trend was evident: energy usage closely correlates with the incidence of seizures.

We had an in-depth discussion about the spreadsheet during our appointment with the internal specialist doctor following the ICU admission. He listened attentively and then posed a question that had not been raised before: "Has anyone suggested a continuous blood glucose monitoring system?"

A simple but significant concept emerged: monitoring blood glucose levels in real time could reveal the key factors triggering seizures.

We left the appointment with a sense of purpose. For the first time, we felt that someone had truly listened and provided a tangible tool to help us navigate the chaos.

That evening, we purchased a continuous glucose monitor (CBGM). It felt like a lifeline—an opportunity to finally collect the data we needed to piece together the puzzle.

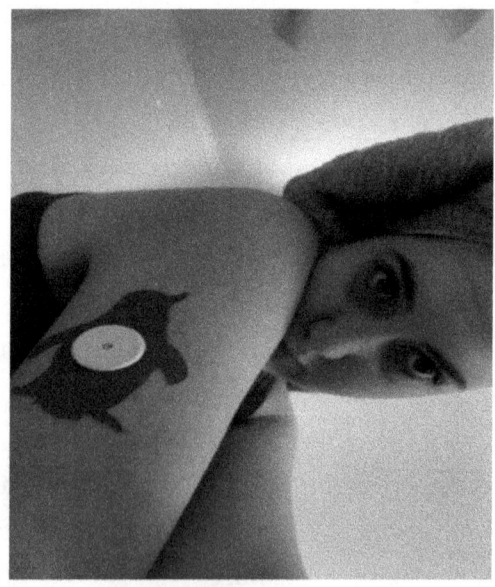

Continuous blood glucose monitor.

The CBGM represented more than just a device; it embodied hope. For the first time, we possessed a tangible tool that could lead us to the answers we had long sought. While our journey continued, we were no longer fumbling in the dark. We were progressing, one step at a time.

A few days later, the CBGM arrived, and we stared at it for the next two days! "What can you tell us?" we eagerly asked. This small, wearable device was designed to deliver real-time information on blood glucose levels, tracking changes around the clock. For the first time, we could monitor something otherwise invisible yet potentially critical.

Just hours after using the CBGM, we noticed unexpected patterns. The data provided a clear insight into Mikayla's bodily internal processes, and it swiftly became evident that something startling was occurring.

A clear pattern soon emerged: blood glucose levels were considerably low and sharply decreased before each seizure. These drops were notably pronounced, occurring suddenly and coinciding with periods of physical stress. Furthermore, we observed a trend related to her workplace; as she spent more time there, increased activity and walking led to a more consistent decline in glucose levels, resulting in a gradual drop over time.

The spreadsheet we meticulously managed aligned perfectly with the CBGM data. High-energy activities, such as long walks, stressful conversations, or intense concentration, appeared to trigger hypoglycaemia. Consequently, seizures ensued.

Overnight readings indicated another concerning trend. Blood glucose levels often dropped to perilously low levels in the early morning hours, despite the absence of seizures. This undetected hypoglycaemia may have been exerting long-term stress on the body, unbeknownst to us.

We provided the CBGM data to the internal specialist, who promptly recognised its significance.

In an instant, everything transformed and became evident.

Fasting prior to the endoscopy and colonoscopy resulted in seizures, necessitating admission to the ICU.

The persistent fatigue we overlooked was likely due to undetected episodes of low blood sugar.

The link between energy consumption and seizures was not merely a hypothesis; solid data now supported our assertion that it was not FND.

Following this new insight, our doctor encouraged Mikayla to continually monitor and log the continuous use of the CBGM to observe trends.

The change was nearly instantaneous. With improved blood sugar management, the seizures not only diminished in frequency and severity but also stopped completely. At last, we felt as though we were regaining control over a situation that had once felt unmanageable.

The CBGM revealed more than merely data; it validated our concerns was about to rectify a misdiagnosis and enhanced our understanding of the seizure's cause. This represented a pivotal moment in our journey, transforming frustration and fear into actionable insights and hope.

Even though we had something tangible, it still didn't elucidate the reason for the decrease in blood glucose. The journey ahead still lay before us, but for the first time, we had a map.

Even with our progress using the CBGM, the mystery lingered. Our internal physician arranged for some tests, and we ended up at Newcastle Private Hospital, where we were expertly cared for by the coronary care and ICU teams and doctors.

The CCU staff treated us as patients and as individuals in need of comfort, compassion, and skilled care. They engaged with Mikayla in a soothing manner, providing reassurance while meticulously monitoring heart rhythms and addressing any immediate issues or risks.

Supported by the ICU doctors during procedures, their expertise is evident, yet their ability to connect with Mikayla was remarkable.

While each test deepened our understanding of the body's internal processes, we could not identify the cause of the blood glucose issue. An endocrinologist was referred for Mikayla. She carefully analysed the data and compared Mikayla's situation to someone stranded in the bush—they can endure 40 consecutive days without food before the body reacts. Mikayla had hardly consumed anything for over 18 months.

She acknowledged that there remained a missing element, which was to determine the reason why she was not eating.

Our endocrinologist recommended a motility gastroenterologist. After nine years at the Mayo Clinic, he had recently resumed his practice in Australia. Renowned for his unyielding curiosity and skill in untangling complex cases, we considered ourselves fortunate to meet with him. The irony was that I had one of his medical journals in my folder.

After evaluating the test results, he had obtained, he called us back into his office. His demeanour was calm yet determined, and we braced for news that could change our lives forever.

At that moment, the confusion and frustration of the past few months—the DIY management plans, the dismissive FND label, and countless hospital visits—seemed to be finally resolving. The tests indicated that a specific gastrointestinal dysfunction was impairing normal digestion.

The results from the two specialists aligned with the AI predictions, both indicating the same two organs. I have securely stored the results in my folder.

Where frustration once prevailed, there now emerged tangible relief—hope strengthened by clear answers and the unwavering commitment of a team. The journey was anything but straightforward; yet, for the first time, we experienced undeniable certainty: we understood the situation and had the right individuals guiding us forward.

The relief was immense. A surge of emotion engulfed us. We walked back to the car and sat in silence. Tears streamed down my face, a mix of exhaustion, relief, and deep gratitude. The burden that had weighed us down for so long began to dissipate, introducing a sense of lightness. This was not the conclusion of our journey, far from it. We had a roadmap, a diagnosis, and a clear plan of action; more than anything, we had hope.

Even amidst this chaos, a feeling of tranquillity emerged that had been absent for quite some time. We embraced a renewed sense of purpose that dispelled the lingering uncertainty and paralysing fear surrounding the unknown.

It wasn't merely about receiving the correct diagnosis; it was about regaining our agency within the medical system, making sure our voices were acknowledged and our concerns addressed seriously.

What unifies this lengthy journey? The doctors who truly listened were instrumental in assisting Mikayla in regaining her health and her entire life. It took five doctors from four different specialties to piece everything together. This was a complex puzzle that a single-organ specialist might overlook – and in fact, did overlook. The body operates as an interconnected machine; therefore, we must adopt this perspective in the diagnostic process. Embracing a holistic view of bodily function is particularly crucial in intricate health circumstances and conditions.

We survived and persevered, emerging stronger and more resilient than ever. Our journey validates the power of hope, resilience, and the enduring strength of family. This narrative is one of struggle, yet it also highlights triumph—reclaiming control amidst overwhelming odds.

Moreover, it serves as both a cautionary tale and a guide for others, emphasising the importance of steadfast advocacy and the right to question medical decisions when something seems amiss.

CHAPTER 24

MIKAYLA AND THE FAMILY TODAY

Can a single word truly encapsulate Mikayla at this moment? Not quite—too many springs to mind too quickly.

It's simpler to describe what she isn't. She is working, not in bed, and is not worn out, frustrated, angry, or suspicious of doctors. The last one may still be evolving. But can I convey the magnitude of the change? Absolutely. She's akin to two individuals—one who is present and another who is a powerful force navigating life.

It's not just Mikayla; the entire family, both immediate and extended, feels the impact. The recovery process has been daunting. We found ourselves just waiting. Is she overexerting herself? Is her recovery enough? Has she built up enough reserves in her body? It took a long time to stop holding my breath every time something thudded to the floor above, echoing down the stairs. One second, two seconds, three seconds. Alright, that's enough. Mikayla, are you okay? Sorry, Mum, I forgot to call out and say that I'm fine. We all understood what those thuds on the floor meant.

I can now hold on for 10 seconds before the panic sets in. My stomach churns, and my palms grow sweaty. It's not that I anticipate her seizing; it's the haunting echo of that sound and everything it signifies. Even the sirens of ambulances racing down our street linger in my thoughts, reminding me of what these families are about to endure.

Initially, a wave of relief washed over us following the final diagnosis, but that emotion gradually faded, supplanted by a muted, disquieting calm. The treatment felt disconnected from the anguish we endured; it was in stark contrast to our ordeal and the turmoil we faced.

The journey also involved emotional healing. Mistrust of doctors, except for those accompanying us, proved challenging. Each time we returned to the hospital grounds, anxiety and anger resurfaced for all of us.

Then there were the public places Mikayla painfully claimed she had not returned to—those we are only now revisiting. These were places she regularly frequented, where laughter and enjoyment occurred.

At the beach, Alana was alone with Mikayla, who suffered multiple seizures on the sand. Alana called for an ambulance while she endeavoured to keep Meeka calm and ensured that Mikayla's face remained clear of the sand.

Mikayla and Alana often took Meeka to this spot to play. Although they have not returned since, it will eventually become part of their "to-do" list.

The gym where Alana was a member is a night we are unlikely to forget. Alana took Mikayla to the gym for some light exercise. Do you remember the mindfulness and exercise advice from the neurologists? This occasion likely provided the clearest connection between energy consumption and seizures.

The call came from Alana. I recognised the words that would follow when I heard her struggle to breathe. I summoned my calm, reassuring tone, despite its inclination to quaver. Where was she? Had the ambulance been called? Was she still having seizures? Yes, yes, and yes were the answers.

"Do you want me to come to you?" "No, we're fine – just meet us at the hospital," she replied. But everything was far from alright. Thirty minutes later, Alana called – the ambulance had stopped on the roadside. "What should I do now?" she asked. "Just wait and observe; let's see how things unfold." Within moments, one ambulance crew had grown into three ambulances with six paramedics, all gathered by the roadside. Mikayla continued to relive the flashbacks from that night in the ambulance, hearing them exclaim, "We are losing her." Neither of them had returned to that gym since.

The financial burden was immense. The costs of treatment, medication, and therapy were exorbitant. Being self-employed also entails losing valuable business time—when the team is left unsupported, decisions are postponed, opportunities are lost, and clients drift away.

Business recovery is not merely about resuming operations; it necessitates time—not just days, but potentially months or even years. We will achieve our goals, but time is the ultimate resource that cannot be recovered or cycled back. Once it is lost, it cannot be retrieved indefinitely.

Although we had health insurance, our out-of-pocket expenses rose rapidly. Constant anxiety, uncertainty regarding the future, and fear of setbacks imposed a heavy burden.

We greatly relied on our network of family and friends, who provided practical assistance, emotional support, and constant reminders that we were not alone in this struggle. We recognised the significance of leaning on those who cared for us, embracing vulnerability, and accepting help. This experience was humbling yet crucial to our journey and survival.

An exceptional psychologist established a nurturing environment for us to explore our emotions, express our fears and frustrations, and confront the trauma we faced.

The ongoing worry and stress strained our relationships with family and friends. Our challenges weighed heavily on them, and their steadfast support was vital to our journey. We needed to learn how to express our needs clearly, request help when necessary, and embrace the support offered. Eventually, we came to understand that seeking assistance was not a sign of weakness, but rather a testament to our strength and resilience.

Where do we stand today? We possess a renewed optimism regarding our future. We're creating joyful memories, enabling us to reflect on those moments and harness them for the greater good. It's not merely about careers or financial rewards in a new position. A significant shift has been our revitalised sense of purpose. We recognised that our experiences could and can aid others, uncovering a profound sense of meaning in utilising our narrative to foster positive change in the healthcare system.

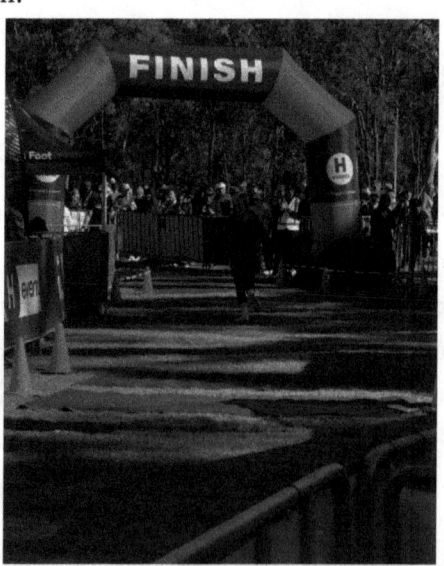

July 2024 Mikayla's first running race.

MUM, PLEASE HELP ME

Over time, we discovered that our scars are not merely reminders of past struggles but powerful symbols of our strength, resilience, and unwavering commitment to achieving a more just and compassionate healthcare system. Our family was transformed—scarred yet stronger—our connections deepened by the trials we shared. We became passionate advocates for patients' rights, devoted to preventing others from enduring similar suffering.

Our renewed goal is to leverage our experience to create change.

CHAPTER 25

RESILIENCE THROUGH COURAGE

The scars are etched into our family's history. They remind us of the pain we endured, the obstacles we confronted, and the lessons we learned. However, they do not define us. Rather, they symbolise our strength, resilience, and unwavering dedication to advocating for justice and improved healthcare for all.

Our journey has transformed us, and we are committed to preventing other families from experiencing the pain and suffering we endured. Our story transcends our struggle; it stands as a call to action, a testament to resilience, and a hopeful reminder that even in the darkest times, light shines through.

MUM, PLEASE HELP ME

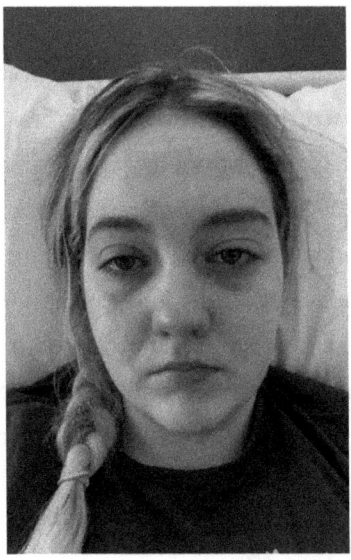

There were days when Mikayla was just so very sad and sick.

This was not our first experience requiring resilience and bravery, both individually and as a family. Our previous experiences have nurtured a deep resilience, enabling us to draw courage from within—an inner strength that inspires others.

In 2004, my life changed drastically, making it difficult to envision my future. Significant events like that indeed transform lives. The fear in your eyes, loss, and internal disappointment are hard to conceal. Gradually, over the years that followed, I started to accept my situation and discovered that living with heart failure was not an end but rather a challenge that inspired me to live life in a new way. I acknowledge that there were many times when I struggled to embrace this perspective. I realised that cherishing each mundane moment was essential to finding peace amid mental turmoil.

It felt like a significant loss. I felt diminished—not only as an individual but also in the value I could contribute to society. How could I succeed if I could not help myself?

We adapted as a family, established a new normal, and moved forward with life. I realised the benefits of outsourcing.

Next came the challenge of being a single parent while building a business. It was no easy task. I faced fatigue and uncertainty, yet my inner strength remained resilient. The encouragement from my children, who had matured into strong and caring individuals, continually reinforced the importance of my strength in their lives.

However, my roar was not solely about its outward effects but also about my inner transformation. I found peace within myself, realising that my life held purpose and significance beyond the challenges I faced. By embracing my roar, I could let go of self-doubt and fear, replacing them with courage and confidence in my abilities. I tackle setbacks with resilience, learning from each experience to strengthen my resolve to succeed. I fiercely protect my dreams, refusing to allow adversity to deter me from the path of my goals.

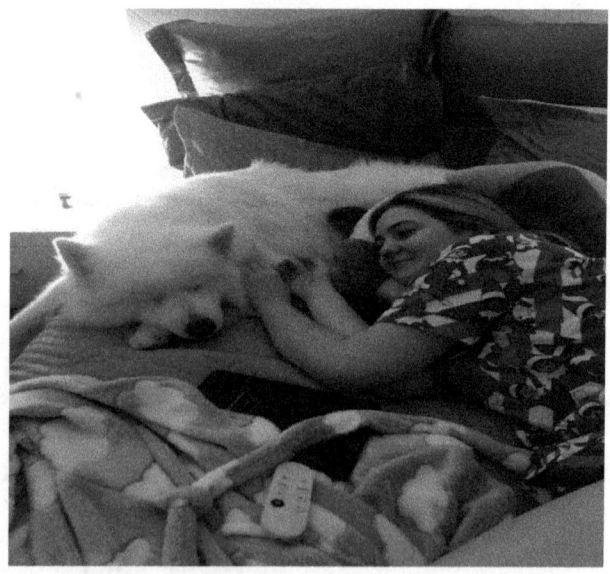

Meeka was by Mikayla's side every day.

Navigating adversity requires a long-term commitment to remaining authentic to one's past and present selves. The feeling of loss is genuine. I recognise that I am not the same individual I was before 2004. Utilising the skills gained from facing challenges and fostering resilience has led to a life that is more meaningful, connected, and empathetic toward others.

My children observed strength, courage, resourcefulness, and joy, even in what others might deem challenging situations. We were a tight-knit family that supported one another and always looked out for each other. Our laughter acted as our medicine, and openness was vital for communication.

This time, however, Mikayla's seizures took us in a different direction. They were intense and unforgiving, resembling an aggressive battle that showed no signs of resolution. We all felt the mounting stress, anxiety, and pervasive fear that lingered in the atmosphere. The children's social lives suffered, and their emotional health declined. They witnessed my struggles, my face marked by worry, and my spirits weighed down by the relentless fight. As a result, they were compelled to mature beyond their years, assuming responsibilities that were far too burdensome for them.

They experienced ongoing frustration, anger, and conflicts with healthcare providers, which left its mark on them.

Despite the chaos, something extraordinary occurred. Faced with overwhelming challenges, our family grew even stronger. The shared struggle against medical negligence forged a deeper bond than we had ever experienced. This connection transcended the personal burdens we each carried. We learned to rely on one another, provide support, and communicate in unprecedented ways. Even new relationships began to form amidst the turmoil and chaos.

We recognised the significance of acknowledging our challenges, validating each other's feelings, and seeking solace in our shared experiences.

We established rituals—small acts of kindness, gestures of support, and shared laughter that pierced through the darkness—to help us navigate the emotional turmoil. We held family meetings that often extended late into the evening, during which we discussed the day's discoveries. We connected to express our feelings and reaffirm our love and commitment to each other.

We held numerous gatherings in the intervention lounge. Often, late at night, it transformed into a sacred space where we could share our anxieties, fears, and hopes without judgment. It became a sanctuary, allowing us to be vulnerable without fear.

The scars from this experience linger, reminding us of the pain, suffering, and challenges we faced together. However, they do not define us. Instead, they symbolise our honour and demonstrate our resilience, unity, and deep love for one another. Our collective journey has strengthened us, transforming us into a more resilient family interconnected by shared experiences.

Through our family's journey, we learned the crucial role of communication, the importance of openly recognising and validating each other's feelings, and the strength of shared resilience. We became skilled at listening, supporting, and relying on each other during our weaker moments. Even in our darkest hours, we realised that family bonds can provide the strength and resilience needed to face seemingly insurmountable obstacles.

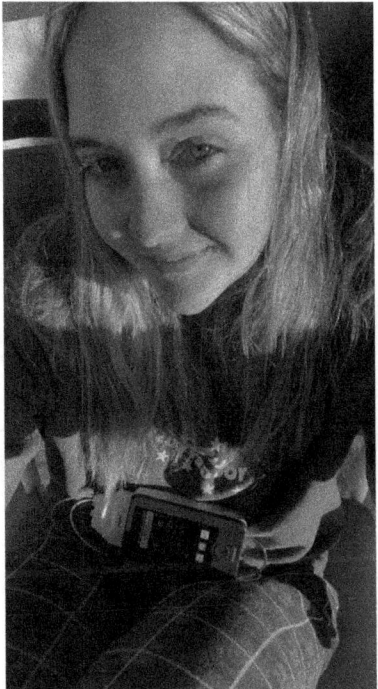

Getting out in the sunshine.

The experience affected our immediate and extended family and friends. Their steadfast support served as a vital lifeline, offering both emotional and practical assistance. Together, they played a significant role in our journey to discover resilience.

The entire experience underscored the essential importance of empowering patients. We acknowledged the need to be informed, assertive, and determined in pursuing optimal care outcomes.

The journey has been challenging, marked by despair and uncertainty, yet also by our unwavering hope and the strength of our family. It continues to shape our lives, altering our understanding of the healthcare system and our relationships with one another.

KAREN PERKS

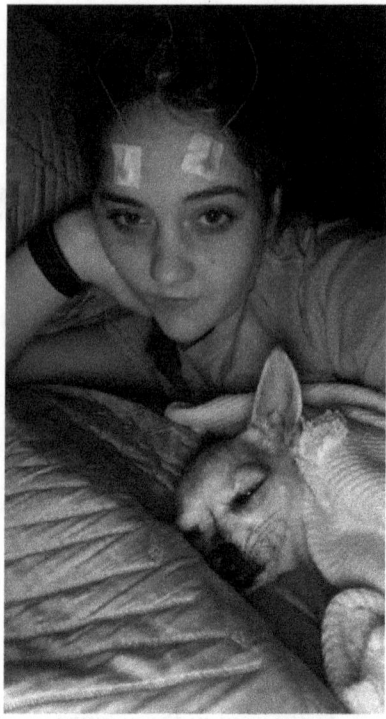

Mikayla was surrounded by love.

Although the experience has been incredibly challenging, it has fostered a remarkable and deeply rewarding strength within our family. It serves as a strong testament to the resilience of the human spirit and the enduring influence of love and family during difficult times. We have all learned to embody even greater resilience, finding effectiveness in our identity and actions. We firmly believe in our capacity to conquer the seemingly impossible through wisdom and gratitude. My insights gained from overcoming challenges have resulted in discoveries and the emergence of a new self.

Be brave. Embrace the new you. Stay true to yourself. Be honest about who you are and don't accept the limitations imposed by others.

CHAPTER 26

BEING GRATEFUL

Gratitude is a powerful force that alters our perception of the world, influences our daily experiences, and impacts our recovery after hardship. As I sit here in reflection, I feel deep gratitude—not merely the temporary, polite kind, but the profound, soul-nourishing version that compels me to stop, breathe, and recognise how fortunate we are.

Above all, I am grateful that Mikayla is alive. This simple truth holds a depth that words cannot express. Life is fragile, and over the past year and a half, I've encountered moments filled with fear, uncertainty, and ambiguity regarding the future. Yet here we are. She is here; that alone brings my heart daily gratitude.

Each laugh, hug, and shared moment reminds me of the value of life. It would be easy to overlook these moments, but I choose not to. Instead, I cherish them, knowing that every day we have together is a blessing. I also appreciate Alana and Reece's different abilities to help and their constant presence for us. Thank you for your unwavering support; I will always be grateful and love you both unconditionally.

I am grateful that we received the correct diagnosis in just 18 months.

While some may consider that a lengthy duration, it is relatively short in the context of medical mysteries. Many individuals endure years, even decades, without clarity. The lengthy wait, unceasing search, and numerous tests and appointments can be exhausting.

Thankfully, we uncovered the truth and mapped our path ahead. This alone is worthy of gratitude, as knowledge empowers us. Understanding our situation enabled us to progress with treatment, care, and hope. Although that journey presented its challenges, it ultimately directed us to where we needed to be. For that, my gratitude knows no bounds.

In a world of uncertainty, I appreciate that we all have jobs. I do not take stability for granted. The opportunity to work, provide for others, and find meaning in our activities offers us comfort and security. I understand that not everyone shares this fortune. Having jobs that sustain us, enable us to care for our families, and encourage planning is a privilege. Although doubts and fears about the future have arisen, we remain present. We stand resilient, continuously progressing, and capable of supporting one another. That is truly a blessing.

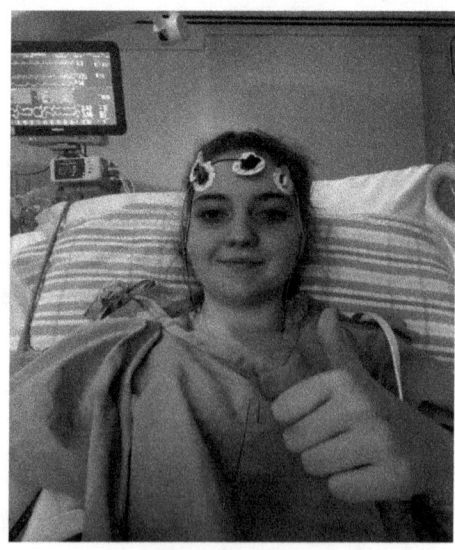

Being grateful.

Throughout this journey, I feared that I might exhaust our family and friends. Watching loved ones bear the burden of medical challenges is incredibly daunting. Yet, despite everything, our community remained steadfast. They offered their support, showered us with love, and never allowed us to feel like a burden. I am profoundly grateful for this.

Times of hardship can strain relationships, yet ours remained resilient. We relied on one another as needed, and somehow, we all emerged stronger instead of depleted. That is truly remarkable. Having a support system that withstands trials, stays unwavering, and offers consistent assistance in tough times is a precious gift I shall always cherish.

Amidst our challenges and achievements, we feel immense gratitude for the opportunity to positively impact others. There is a profound sense of fulfilment in giving back, sharing our stories, and supporting those who share a similar journey. Our struggles mould us, educate us, and provide us with insights that allow us to connect meaningfully with others. I do not merely wish to endure this journey; I aim to leverage it to assist others. Providing comfort, guidance, or simply an empathetic ear to someone in need is what drives me.

I am grateful for the opportunity to learn about the procedures and systems within the healthcare profession. Understanding their operations, acquiring knowledge, and navigating complexities has proven invaluable. This experience has provided me with insights, skills, and a greater appreciation for the frameworks that support us. The knowledge I've gained will remain with me, aiding my future endeavours and enabling me to assist others in similar situations.

I sincerely appreciate the close circle of people who assisted me in finding the right doctors. Obtaining proper medical care isn't always straightforward, and having trustworthy individuals to guide me with recommendations and insights made a significant difference. Their support saved time, reduced stress, and helped us identify the right solutions. I will always value such assistance and guidance.

Above all, I appreciate faith – that steadfast conviction that I would not be alone. Faith supported me during my most challenging times, reassuring me that I was not forsaken even in my bleakest moments. Through prayer, hope, or the gentle reassurance that everything would be all right, faith served as my anchor. It provided stability, reminding me of a broader plan and a more significant perspective than I could currently perceive. Faith manifests in various ways.

Life is not always a smooth journey; it presents challenges, heartbreak, and moments of uncertainty. However, gratitude anchors me and highlights what truly matters, redirecting my attention from losses to gains, fear to hope, and doubt to appreciation. Each day offers a chance to embrace gratitude, acknowledge the beauty in even the most challenging experiences, and cherish the elements that make life worthwhile.

The future is uncertain for us all, but gratitude will remain my guiding force. It acts as a reminder to celebrate small successes, cherish the friends who support me, and value every moment. Life and love are priceless. Today, as I write at the kitchen bench, I feel an immense gratitude for everything.

CHAPTER 27

THANK YOU TO YOU

Kindness is a gift generally given without expecting anything in return. When received, it is cherished so deeply that the giver remains in your thoughts. The recipient often recounts the story with joy, enthusiasm, and gratitude. You may not remember their name, and although their face may fade, their impact on your life at that moment will always resonate with you.

Amidst the darkness, we encountered angels who were placed in our way to uplift us. Clad in uniforms, scrubs, and ties, these remarkable individuals brightened our days, enabling us to smile authentically and laugh heartily, all while feeling secure under their care. Their compassion transformed our emotions, allowing us to make wise choices and plans with a calm and reassured mindset. They were not kind out of obligation—they were genuinely considerate people. What a gem to discover amid the chaos.

AMBULANCE PARAMEDICS

We encountered many of them. Initially, there was one ambulance with two paramedics during the first few visits. Soon enough, this changed to two ambulances with three or four paramedics. By Christmas, we warmly opened the front door, greeting them with, "How are you?" and "Great to see you again." There were playful invitations to join us for Christmas lunch as we stood side by side, waiting for the fire and rescue team to safely bring Mikayla down the stairs, unconscious and connected to tubes.

We discussed her symptoms and our progress, being patient with Meeka, who would try to jump into the ambulance with Mikayla, sensing that something was amiss. She would lie quietly beside Mikayla, always by her side.

NURSE AT ED

One night, when we needed a bit of extra kindness, a lovely, confident, and experienced nurse appeared at Resus Bed 2. She had flowers in her hair and was well-acquainted with the ED. We watched as Mikayla had a seizure, gently stroking her hair, ensuring her body didn't hit the steel bars of the bed, and adjusting the pillows to the best position.

My concerns about the spreadsheet are being ignored yet again. I felt as though I had been transported back to school, where the teacher, brimming with confidence, insists they are correct while I, the student, plead for a chance to clarify how this complex tool operates. Scolded and labelled as troublesome, I was dismissed to the naughty corner.

The doctor turned and walked away, prompting me to lower my head. I felt the amazing nurse's presence close by as she encouraged me, "Just keep going—you are on the right path." I asked, "Can't you tell the doctor?" She replied, "Just keep going," and then she disappeared. So, I carried on.

DOCTOR IN ED

He was patient and compassionate, leaving his ego at the door. Mikayla's doctor, on two occasions, dedicated time to clarify the limitations while advocating for her treatment—striving to keep her in the emergency department rather than transferring her unconscious to a poorly staffed, dim ward in the middle of the night. Several times, I opposed the neurologists' approach, which stemmed from the belief that there was nothing more they could do. I argued that it contravened their procedures and referenced their public documents. I sought ways to protect my daughter from harm, warned the neurologists, and vowed to do everything within my power to prevent any danger to her.

On those two separate nights, I felt assured of her safety; I could return home for a shower and a brief rest, confident that she was in capable hands with him.

MCDONALD'S TEAM

These kids achieved something remarkable. Their relationships with their Macca peers should be admired in any workplace. Armed with straightforward instructions on what to do, how to do it, and when to do it, they consistently supported their colleagues. "Kazza," they would say, "she has fallen." This is our cue for everyone to pitch in.

Some may have misinterpreted the group pictures with Mikayla on the floor, yet the bond among that close-knit team was unbreakable. They didn't rise to the occasion out of obligation or job title; they did so to support their friend from a genuine desire.

GENERAL PRACTITIONER (GP)

Our GP accompanied us on this journey. He felt the pressure during the tough times, especially the most challenging moments. Nonetheless, his outstanding contribution was his trust in my understanding of Mikayla. He believed I would never compromise her safety and recognised the complexity of the situation. He comprehended that overcoming it required teamwork.

OUR FIRST INTERNAL PHYSICIAN

With remarkable wisdom and compassion, he was the first physician to decisively dismiss FND. He approached Mikayla patiently and methodically, and I appreciated listening to their discussions about the complexities of various conditions. He guided us accurately, yet it's disheartening how some doctors disregarded his experience and seniority, labelling him as if he were on a fishing expedition. Well, he almost succeeded in catching the fish.

OUR SECOND INTERNAL PHYSICIAN

We encountered this doctor after Mikayla was admitted to the ICU due to seizures following anaesthesia from day surgery. I presented my spreadsheet to him, and he enquired, "Has anyone recommended checking your blood glucose levels?" He also suggested using a continuous blood glucose monitor to track fluctuations. What was the result? We identified an issue, and since then, Mikayla has only seized during planned tests.

ENDOCRINOLOGIST

The first endocrinologist we met in the ED, it took 45 minutes for her to deliver a diagnosis. However, her diagnosis was left in the patient records. No further action was taken. The patient discharge papers were not completed and never received.

The second endocrinologist we met privately, and she provided the same diagnosis.

MOTILITY GASTROENTEROLOGIST

Investigating the cause of Mikayla's low blood glucose, initially triggered by nausea while eating. The highly skilled doctor, who had spent nine years at the Mayo Clinic, also authored several medical journals in my expanding collection. After a 45-minute discussion, we left with a possible explanation and subsequently a diagnosis. He was extremely knowledgeable, compassionate, and innovative.

PRIVATE HOSPITAL

This has never been a public or private debate. Instead, it involved a team of compassionate, open-minded healthcare professionals who listened to Mikayla and me, exceeding our expectations. This experience highlights how patient-centred care results in remarkable outcomes. We thank all the doctors and nurses in Coronary Care and ICU.

MY TEAM

On a personal level, I would like to sincerely thank my team across various countries. Your support, your attentiveness, and your patience are forever appreciated.

OUR NEIGHBOURS

Sometimes, they managed traffic control, while at other times, they keep an eye on our dogs. They are genuinely kind and sincere, traits anyone would wish for in a neighbour.

PART SIX

CHAPTER 28

THE IMPORTANCE OF HAVING YOUR PATIENT RECORDS

It is extremely difficult to understand how to navigate and advocate for them. We faced challenges with Mikayla's records. Efforts to gather patient information were met with obstacles, scepticism, and even claims that we couldn't have the information and that we couldn't grasp it. We were informed that the doctors were too busy to help us, stating that they alone could interpret or read the records since we wouldn't comprehend them.

As a result, we organised the symptoms into our central database and compiled our own records. We managed to collect medical journals and summarise data – we accomplished it all except obtaining Mikayla's medical records.

Healthcare has evolved, with one of the most transformative shifts being the move towards patients having full access to their health records, except for Australia.

The Health Insurance Portability and Accountability Act (HIPAA) stipulates that patients must be allowed to review and amend their medical records. I know this because I downloaded the legislation and took it to the hospital, only to be told I had misread it. By this point, I was accustomed to being gaslighted and recognised the necessity of having evidence for any discussions. And how dare they claim that! I understood this act better than the hospital staff did. But imagine if you, as a patient or carer, had no experience with legislation. How do you defend your rights? It is unlikely – they are a forceful bunch.

We strongly advocate for patients to have access to all their records, not just referral letters and a handful of blood test results, but also detailed information.

We know from experience the benefits it would have offered to those interested in assisting – Mikayla's GP and the internal physicians. The medical professionals recognised that they were acting as detectives. How can you solve a problem without having most, or even some, of the information?

Traditionally, medical records have been confined to hospital systems, clinics, and doctors' offices, accessible only to healthcare professionals. However, research highlighted by another medical journal indicates that when patients can directly access their medical records, they gain a deeper understanding of their health status. This knowledge empowers them to take proactive steps in managing their wellbeing.

Access to medical records allows patients to make informed choices about their treatment options, lifestyle decisions, and overall healthcare journey. Comprehending past diagnoses, prescribed medications, and test results enables patients to ask insightful questions, engage in shared decision-making, and take charge of their health.

But what if you are unwell and unable to obtain answers? This information is critical, and you have the right to access it. It is not a matter of desire; it is a priority and a necessity.

Our schoolteachers instruct us from a young age that knowledge is power. This principle profoundly applies to healthcare. Patients know their bodies best. Mikayla understood her body well and had valuable insights into her symptoms and experiences. We documented this knowledge in a well-known spreadsheet and graphs, but nobody at the hospital took the time to examine it.

It is logical that a patient who can provide a complete and updated medical history reduces the risk of information gaps. When doctors have access to accurate and comprehensive information, continuity of care is enhanced, and clinical decision-making becomes more effective. This principle applies to all professions where someone gives advice. You need the complete history to be informed. In medicine, the consequences are far more severe.

The benefit is that physicians no longer rely solely on patient recollections, which may be incomplete or inaccurate. Instead, they can examine comprehensive records, including laboratory results, imaging reports, allergies, previous treatments, and medication histories.

Strengthened doctor-patient trust and communication

Medical records often include complex terminology and clinical notes that may be challenging for patients to understand. Here is an intriguing concept: why not allow the patient to determine what they need explained?

The expansion of electronic health records (EHRs), patient portals, and mobile health applications is accelerating worldwide. Many healthcare systems are implementing policies that encourage transparency, data sharing, and patient empowerment – except in Australia.

As healthcare continues to evolve, the future should adopt a more collaborative model in which patients and doctors collaborate with a shared understanding of health data. Eliminating barriers to information ensures that healthcare becomes more personalised, efficient, and ultimately more effective for all stakeholders involved.

KAREN PERKS

In Mikayla's case, even a delay of seven days was too lengthy given the swift progression of her cluster of seizures. More than twelve months have now passed, and we are still waiting – that is outrageous.

CHAPTER 29

EIGHT SPECIALTIES AND COUNTING

Mikayla's journey through the healthcare system was exhausting. She consulted eight specialties, each offering its perspective—but never the complete picture. Each time, it felt as though she was starting afresh, explaining her symptoms repeatedly in the hope that someone would finally connect the dots. I had the spreadsheet—they could have looked at that—and it contained all the connections, complete with graphs.

But instead of answers, there was frustration, lost in a maze of disconnected opinions. The result? It became a fragmented experience where crucial pieces of her story were overlooked, leaving her without the clarity she desperately needed.

THE SPECIALISTS SHE SAW

- Cardiology – The first few presentations to the ED exhibited cardiac and neurological symptoms. However, this revealed a pattern – each time she experienced a seizure, her heart rate would spike dramatically until the seizure subsided.

- Neurology – They were there at the start – please offer a consultation. Then they took over like a disease, tentacles sprawling throughout the hospital with their FND diagnosis.
- Psychology – Referred by the neurologists, the best they could offer was a fear of vomiting. Well, who doesn't have that? Nutrition – Missed opportunity – although they addressed the lack of food with liquid replacements, they didn't consider why she wasn't eating. Instead, they focused on making her eat more.
- Gastroenterology – There were five gastroenterologists in total– only one got it right, and it took 45 minutes. One, with his deadpan bedside manner, diagnosed constipation, and another diagnosed functional gut syndrome. Both were wrong. But it is not about them being incorrect – it was about they didn't listen. Didn't stop to consider they may be missing something.
- Endocrinology – These were the only specialists who made the correct diagnosis the first time – one from the public and one from the private systems. Both were female doctors.
- ICU (Intensive Care Unit) – The doctor listened and understood that there was something in my spreadsheet, so he referred me to the admitting specialist. Back to neurology, we go, and nothing changes.

THE DEPARTMENTS SHE DIDN'T SEE

- Maternity (Obstetrics & Gynaecology)
- Orthopaedics
- Paediatrics
- Oncology (Cancer)

Apart from the obvious reasons these specialties were not investigated, the point is that she continued to be passed around the siloed specialties, meeting a new doctor with each admission.

When a patient moves between specialists without finding a resolution, the issue often lies not in a lack of expertise but in a lack of coordination. The medical system is designed to diagnose in silos, yet complex cases require collaboration across specialties. This was the chief challenge for Mikayla.

CHAPTER 30

BUT WHY DID THIS HAPPEN?

Is the system broken? Or have we tried to be too clever and delve deeply into single-organ medicine and specialties? One thing is clear: the absence of dedicated case management or general medicine as a specialty within the hospital significantly contributed to the breakdown in Mikayla's patient care, particularly concerning her complex multi-system illnesses.

In a hospital system where specialties dominate, and no single discipline is responsible for coordinating care across various areas, patients with complex or undiagnosed conditions can easily fall through the cracks.

But this wasn't the real reason – she was misdiagnosed, and the neurologists simply unequivocally refused to look beyond the initial FND diagnosis, even as the patient continuously provided data indicating her symptoms were worsening.

Is this a cultural issue or an issue of arrogance and stubbornness, characterised by an inability to recognise that others have a role equal to that of the doctor? When reviewing the specialty that succeeded twice – once in the public hospital and once in the private sector – both instances involved female doctors. Does this also suggest a gender issue?

Although specialists are experts in their fields, they may lack the training or time to recognise and address conditions that affect multiple organs or systems. No one asks them to be God. Internal medicine practitioners are trained to identify when a case falls outside the scope of a single specialty and to consult with other specialists. They serve as the glue that binds the medical team together, ensuring that all aspects of a patient's health are addressed.

When we shared the investigation strategies of our internal medicine specialists with the neurologists, they dismissed them as merely a "fishing expedition." Is there a hierarchy among the specialties? At least the internal medicine specialists were trying to investigate. Trying to find an answer.

I asked several times where patients with complex medical diagnoses go – we were informed that there is no provision for them in this hospital, and that those experiencing seizures are referred to neurology.

Hospitals can address these issues by formalising internal medicine as a core specialty, enhancing case management, improving care coordination, and reducing diagnostic errors. A holistic, patient-centred approach encompassing comprehensive oversight and interdisciplinary collaboration is essential for a functioning healthcare system that meets the needs of all patients. Although it is too late for these changes to assist Mikayla, hopefully, no 18-year-old will have to endure the same journey in the future.

CHAPTER 31

THE FINANCIAL COST IS TO EVERYBODY

Nobody contemplates the financial cost of medical misdiagnosis or negligence until they are amidst it. It impacts not just the person with an undiagnosed or misdiagnosed illness but forms a web that extends and grows. The web does not stop until it is dismantled. Does the cost ever stop? Not really. It just reduces to a trickle that forever drains the funder.

I knew the web was present and expanding because we review figures each week. I also realised this because I spent more time at the hospital than a full-time employee. When you can stroll down the corridors and recognise a staff member well enough to greet them with a "Hi, how are you?", it indicates you are spending too much time in a hospital. Or when the ambulance paramedics know us by name and joke about having Christmas lunch together, then it's clear there is a problem.

The apparent players—Mikayla, Alana, Reece, and me—are the immediate family. Even Meeka, our dog, was affected. The financial impact resonates like a tsunami to stakeholders who are never considered.

You can almost sing Mikayla's government-funded resource list to the tune of The Twelve Days of Christmas.

On the first day of Christmas there were ...

- 35+ ambulances
- 60+ paramedics
- 25 ED doctors
- Nurses (too many to count)
- One x patient transfer between hospitals
- One x fire and rescue
- Three x public hospitals
- Two x private hospitals
- One GP
- Two internal specialists
- Eight neurologists
- Six+ radiologists
- Two x nutritionists
- Two x psychologists,
- Four gastroenterologists, and
- Two endocrinologists – the two female specialists who diagnosed the first part correctly the first time and linked it to an underlying GI health issue.

Other expenses for the public and private health systems include:

- Food and beverage (not really for Mikayla as she was barely eating)

- Cleaning
- Medication
- Private health insurance providers
- Administration staff

and I am confident this is not the end of the list.

I cannot even begin to assign a dollar value to the public health cost of misdiagnosis. If these resources are required for just one person, imagine the financial burden on taxpayers across every state if thousands of individuals are either undiagnosed or misdiagnosed. These hospitals receive partial funding from the Commonwealth. You may not have experienced long-term illness and may think it is not your concern, but undiagnosed and misdiagnosed conditions affect us all.

The financial impact is even greater than these costs. The figures mentioned represent the direct expenses necessary to address immediate medical needs. Beyond this, there is the financial implication of adding further resources to accommodate the influx of car accidents, heart attacks, strokes, other illnesses, and a myriad of additional medical demands that continuously arise.

Mikayla's use of resources halted their deployment elsewhere. Have you ever explained a comprehensive financial impact model to doctors to encourage them to increase their efforts? It involves explaining that funds and resources are being wasted due to the inaccurate diagnosis of her condition. In my experience, it's not worth the effort.

If funding is not provided to address other patient needs, there is one reason for a full waiting room. At times, I felt guilty knowing there was another cause, yet we continued to experience "Groundhog Day" in the emergency department. If they had truly listened and diagnosed correctly… Well, that is another discussion.

The financial burden on our family was substantial. When you hear the phrase, "it is expensive to be sick," think of a figure and then multiply it by 20, and you will be close. The longer you remain unwell, the greater that number will be. For us, the figure was as follows.

Mikayla: Loss of income for 18 months; loss of two full-time positions – she had functional neurological disorder (FND) noted on her medical records and had been prescribed psychiatric medication for the gastrointestinal issue.

Alana: Costs associated with psychology, unpaid leave when taking sick leave, and other direct expenses incurred while at the hospital – such as parking, coffee, and hospital cafés.

Karen: GP fees, out of pocket for all private specialists, procedures, tests, parking, hospital cafés, and psychologists. All household functions were outsourced. Additionally, there was the financial impact on the business – hundreds of thousands of dollars in lost revenue each year; all staff positions were made redundant, resulting in financial loss for them too – where is this accounted for? Loss of new project opportunities ensued. International growth halted.

So how much did it cost this family and anyone associated? Nearly $1,000,000. The emotional scars and frustrations cannot be quantified economically. We accept these as opportunities for personal growth, character building, courage, and resilience – allocated somewhere in the ledger of life.

PART SEVEN

CHAPTER 32

EVOLUTION OF THE MEDICAL PROFESSION

To understand where to begin advocating for yourself, you need to understand how these monolithic organisations called public hospitals have evolved to work as they do now.

This section of the forthcoming chapters focuses on reflection—specifically on an industry, a profession—a critically important profession that can save lives and cause loss of life if not properly managed. Our path forward relies on reflecting on the history of the medical profession and questioning why such organisations fail their customers, the patients. It is also essential to recognise that hospitals operate like businesses; they have procedures, policies, and minimum standards. Simplifying the complex will help others navigate challenges like those we have faced.

This is not a criticism – you cannot change the past, only influence the future. Reflect on the past and use that reflection to create something better, fairer, and more powerful for good.

After spending hours in the emergency department, cardiology, and neurology and others, I observed interactions between doctors and nurses, between doctors, nurses, and patients, and between doctors, nurses, and family members. Each interaction was unique, shaped by culture and societal norms. However, change is on the horizon, with an expectation that doctors, nurses, patients, and family members will all stand as equals, driven by the rapid advancement of technology. All are motivated by the same goals yet are currently separated by a group striving to cling to the past.

To understand why we are where we are today, we must grasp how the medical profession has developed. This evolution involves an industry long dominated by men, esteemed yet now ensnared in a fanciful world of make-believe shaped by historical, cultural, and social influences. The number of women coming through as doctors is increasing, however it is time before they are in senior positions, specialists, and other influential positions within healthcare.

It is widely recognised that in prehistoric and ancient practices, healing and caregiving frequently assumed communal or family-based roles, with women typically serving as midwives, herbalists, and caregivers.

As societies advanced, the Institutionalisation of medicine and healing practices became formal. In ancient civilisations such as Greece, Rome, and Egypt, men, often educated in philosophy and science, became physicians. Figures such as Hippocrates and Galen established medicine as a scholarly and systematic discipline, primarily accessible to men.

History shows that cultural and religious norms often restricted, and sometimes excluded, women from formal education and leadership positions. In medieval Europe, the professionalisation of healing sidelined women, confining them to roles such as midwifery or exposing them to accusations of witchcraft if they practised outside societal boundaries.

During the Renaissance and Enlightenment, medicine became more closely linked to science. Universities and medical schools appeared as centres of learning, although they largely remained accessible only to men, and the profession of medicine began to develop.

From the Renaissance onwards, medicine became associated with formal education and credentialing due to the emergence of medical schools, which were primarily accessible to wealthy or elite men. Women were barred from entering medical schools or obtaining credentials.

By the 18th and 19th centuries, professional associations and licensing systems established medicine as a career that required institutional approval, marginalising informal healers, many of whom were women.

During the Enlightenment, medicine became linked with science and progress, enhancing its societal status. In alignment with these developments, male doctors acquired authority as experts.

As scientific medicine gained prominence, traditional practices, particularly those led by women, such as midwifery, were devalued or assimilated into male-dominated medical institutions.

Cultural views associated men with leadership, authority, and intellectual pursuits, aligning them with physicians' evolving role as decision-makers.

Although caregiving roles like nursing have become feminised, the more authoritative functions of diagnosing and treating patients continue to be male dominated.

Milestones in medicine, such as eradicating diseases and performing complex surgeries, have elevated doctors' societal status and have had a significant historical impact.

Doctors have historically maintained control over knowledge, terminology, and decision-making, creating an atmosphere of exclusivity and authority. Throughout history, challenging doctors was socially discouraged due to their perceived expertise and the trust placed in their life-saving skills.

While the gender imbalance in medicine has changed in many areas, with an increasing number of women entering the profession, the historical legacy of male dominance and societal reverence for doctors continues to influence perceptions of authority and trustworthiness in the field.

Historically, the gender imbalance in the medical profession has reinforced a hierarchical structure in which male-dominated roles, such as doctors, are viewed as more authoritative than female-dominated roles, like nursing. This hierarchy stems from social, cultural, and professional factors that have perpetuated disparities in status, power, and decision-making within healthcare.

REINFORCEMENT OF GENDERED ROLES

Until recently, doctors were predominantly men. As universities opened more positions to female students and students from CALD backgrounds, as well as those of Aboriginal or Torres Strait Islander descent, there was limited cultural diversity in the workforce. Consequently, this resulted in limited cultural diversity for patients, as well as potential misogyny for female patients. The increasing number of women entering medicine challenges traditional hierarchies, although barriers to leadership persist.

Historically, men were seen as decision-makers and intellectual leaders, while women were relegated to caregiving and supportive roles. This cultural perception linked doctors with leadership and authority, while associating nurses with nurturing and subordination.

Nursing, which emphasises patient care and emotional support, has been feminised and undervalued compared to the male-dominated, science-oriented "curative" role of doctors.

In healthcare settings, doctors are frequently regarded as leaders of medical teams. They make vital decisions, while nurses execute them, reinforcing a hierarchical structure.

Although nurses play a vital role in patient care, they are often expected to adhere to doctors' orders, which undermines their professional autonomy and influence.

INTERDISCIPLINARY COLLABORATION

Modern healthcare increasingly values team-based approaches, recognising the complementary roles of nurses and other professionals, including doctors.

Historically, the gender imbalance has perpetuated a hierarchy that places male-dominated roles in authority over their female counterparts. Although progress is being made to tackle these inequities, overcoming deeply rooted societal norms and systemic barriers remains vital for establishing a more equitable and collaborative healthcare system.

The hierarchical structure within healthcare, influenced by gender imbalances, may result in medical misdiagnoses stemming from communication barriers, the undervaluation of nursing expertise, and an excessive reliance on traditional power dynamics.

Suppression of input from nurses

Due to their constant presence at the bedside, nurses frequently notice subtle changes in a patient's condition. However, in hierarchical systems, their insights can be undervalued or overlooked, leading to delays in critical diagnoses or interventions.

In rigid hierarchies, there is a **lack of collaborative decision-making.** Decisions are mainly made by doctors, potentially excluding valuable input from nurses and other members of the healthcare team.

This can result in blind spots during diagnostic processes.

Nurses, particularly in male-dominated medical teams, may be reluctant to challenge or question doctors' assessments because they fear reprisal, dismissal, or harm to workplace relationships.

Hierarchical systems often promote a top-down approach, where information flows from doctors to nurses but not vice versa. This can result in the overlooking of critical observations or alternative perspectives.

OVER-RELIANCE ON AUTHORITY

The cultural perception of doctors as the ultimate authority with doctor-centric diagnoses can foster overconfidence in their conclusions, even when evidence suggests alternative possibilities. This respect for authority may impede second opinions or collaborative reassessments.

In a hierarchical structure, the contributions of team members, such as nurses, are often underutilised for multidisciplinary input and are frequently undervalued, limiting the diversity of perspectives that could enhance or correct a diagnosis.

GENDER DYNAMICS AND BIAS

Female nurses, often perceived as occupying subordinate roles, may be stereotyped as lacking clinical expertise. This bias can lead to their observations being dismissed as emotional or unscientific, even when they are clinically relevant.

Female doctors may face challenges in asserting their authority within a male-dominated hierarchy, which can lead to delayed or incorrect diagnoses if their expertise is called into question.

MY OBSERVATION

We observed this countless times in the hospital. The positive but fleeting moments were when the nurse in the ED whispered in my ear to "keep going you are on the right track" and the instance when the female specialist was overlooked by her male counterpart, which subsequently prolonged the diagnostic process. These were two small but impactful moments that supported us on our journey.

Time-sensitive decisions

Nurses often recognise early warning signs of deteriorating patient conditions, yet hierarchical delays in expressing concerns can result in misdiagnoses or delayed treatment. These hierarchies can suppress questioning of decisions made by senior staff, reducing the opportunity to spot errors before they impact patient outcomes.

Research suggests that healthcare systems with more flexible hierarchies and a greater emphasis on interdisciplinary collaboration encounter lower rates of diagnostic errors and enhanced patient outcomes.

Examples of misdiagnoses

High-profile cases of medical errors, documented in the courts, often highlight failures in communication between doctors and nurses as contributing factors, emphasising the dangers of neglecting team input.

The hierarchical structure in healthcare, based on historical and gendered dynamics, can perpetuate medical misdiagnoses by inhibiting communication, undervaluing nursing expertise, and excessively relying on doctors' authority.

Addressing these issues necessitates promoting a culture of collaboration, reducing hierarchies, and acknowledging the essential contributions of all healthcare professionals to patient care.

Parent and caregivers

The exclusion of input from parents and caregivers in healthcare settings, often exacerbated by hierarchical structures, can significantly contribute to medical misdiagnoses. Parents and caregivers hold vital, firsthand information about the patient's symptoms, behaviours, and medical history; however, their voices may be undervalued or overlooked in decision-making processes.

Parents and caregivers, especially those responsible for children, elderly individuals, or patients with disabilities, possess in-depth knowledge of the patient and often observe symptoms and patterns over time that may not be immediately apparent during a clinical visit. They can provide insights into the patient's environment, lifestyle, and responses to previous treatments, which offer vital context and are essential for an accurate diagnosis.

When clinicians ignore observations, they may miss vital contextual cues, leading to inaccurate or incomplete outcome assessments and contributing to misdiagnosis.

Hierarchical communication barriers

Parents and caregivers might feel intimidated or believe their input is unwelcome in a doctor-centric hierarchy, especially if they face dismissive attitudes from healthcare professionals.

Systems that prioritise physician-led decision-making often lack formal mechanisms to incorporate caregiver information into the diagnostic process.

This exclusion raises the possibility and impact of misdiagnoses, especially in complex cases where symptoms are intermittent or subtle atypical.

Bias and stereotyping

Caregivers can be seen as lacking medical expertise, and their input may be dismissed as that of a layperson. This may lead clinicians to underestimate their insights, particularly when caregivers' observations contradict initial clinical impressions.

Mothers, frequently the main caregivers, may face gender biases through gendered dynamics that further undermine the perceived validity of their concerns.

Impact on misdiagnosis

Caregivers might disregard warnings about early or unusual symptoms, resulting in delayed, accurate diagnoses or inappropriate treatment.

Critical information gaps

In many cases, information provided by caregivers about previous treatments, medications, or coexisting conditions is either overlooked during the transfer of information or not communicated effectively, leading to insufficient documentation.

MY OBSERVATION

The gaps in critical information regarding previous treatments were the primary reason we requested access to Mikayla's patient records. We aimed to assist our GP and internal specialist in identifying these gaps and understand the reasoning behind the doctors' decisions, in hopes of establishing any clues. Our intention was never to use that information against them; it was always to aid Mikayla by providing any missing pieces of the puzzle and to address the fragmented care that was occurring.

When patients consult multiple providers, or in hospitals where they are seen by several doctors, the lack of caregiver input can result in fragmented records and overlooked critical connections between symptoms and underlying conditions.

Without a thorough understanding of the patient's history, the consequences of misdiagnosis may occur when healthcare providers overlook patterns, leading to errors or omissions.

There are many solutions, and some, such as technology overhauls, are considered too complex. However, even the simplest changes can have an impact and should be considered for short-term implementation. This problem is not going away, and not doing anything only prolongs positive change.

Cultural and systemic challenges

In diverse populations, linguistic differences or cultural norms may prevent caregivers from expressing their concerns with confidence. Overburdened healthcare systems may not afford caregivers sufficient time to relay detailed observations.

Impact on misdiagnosis

These systemic issues exacerbate communication breakdowns, particularly in fast-paced or high-pressure settings like emergency departments.

Solutions to improve inclusion

Structured feedback mechanisms, when implemented as standardised tools like caregiver questionnaires or pre-visit surveys, can effectively capture essential observations.

Promoting shared decision-making models that actively involve caregivers in discussions about diagnosis and treatment fosters collaborative decision-making.

Training for healthcare professionals: Educating clinicians on the importance of caregiver input and addressing biases that may lead to dismissive attitudes.

Technology integration: Employing patient portals and digital tools to empower caregivers in providing thorough health histories and symptom logs.

Excluding parents and caregivers from the diagnostic process poses significant risks of medical misdiagnosis as it overlooks essential information. Addressing this issue requires systemic changes to promote collaboration, prioritise caregiver input, and foster healthcare environments that value the contributions of all stakeholders in a patient's care.

CHAPTER 33

WHY DO ORGANISATIONS LIKE HEALTHCARE FAIL US?

Why have our hospitals and healthcare failed us, or continue to fail many of us? Lawyers have dedicated medical negligence teams worldwide, which would not be the case if only a few errors or accidents occurred. Their presence is enough to provide a guide to indicate the economic benefit to the lawyers for assisting people with medical negligence claims and hence the number of claims that are being made. The reality is far from utopia.

We understand how we got here and potential solutions to begin changing. However, there are deeper considerations about why healthcare fails us.

Are we overthinking the problems, too afraid to acknowledge that they are of our own making? Blaming others is easier than reflecting on ourselves. Doctors can misuse their technical abilities; however, why does it take so long to address negligent behaviour? Are we back to the same issue of doctors being regarded as untouchable?

MEDICAL KNOWLEDGE AS POWER

Historically, medical knowledge was inaccessible to the public. Access to information about health was limited to a select few professionals, leaving patients largely uninformed about their medical conditions. Medical books, research, and a fundamental understanding of anatomy and diseases were reserved for doctors and specialists. This established a scenario where patients had no choice but to trust their doctors implicitly. Medical professionals were seen as experts in their field and as arbiters of life and death.

In this system, patients rarely questioned their doctors or sought second opinions. The power imbalance between doctor and patient was absolute. Healthcare was not a partnership; it was a service rendered by an authority figure who knew what was best, based on their specialised knowledge.

We recognise how this historical authority was connected to a paternalistic model of care, in which doctors assumed the role of parental figures, making decisions for their patients without their active participation. The paternalistic model maintained that doctors, due to their expertise, were best positioned to make decisions concerning the patient's health, often shielding them from uncomfortable truths or challenging situations.

Patients were often instructed on what to do without being fully informed about the implications of their decisions. This model worked to some extent because many medical conditions had precise, definitive treatments, and patients had limited access to alternative information. However, it rested on the assumption that doctors' judgments were invariably correct, and that patients' opinions were secondary—if they were considered.

KAREN PERKS

THE RISE OF TECHNOLOGY AND INFORMATION ACCESSIBILITY

The internet and digital technology have revolutionised not only the way people communicate, but also how they access information, including healthcare knowledge. The rise of online resources, such as health websites, forums, and peer-reviewed research, has democratised medical information, enabling the public to educate themselves about conditions, treatments, and emerging trends in health issues.

THE INTERNET AS A DOUBLE-EDGED SWORD

While this enhanced access to information has empowered patients, it has also introduced complications. On one hand, patients can now research their own symptoms, gain a deeper understanding of their conditions, and even find alternative treatment options. They can become informed advocates for their own care, seeking out second opinions and engaging more actively with their healthcare providers.

On the other hand, the vast amount of medical information available online is not always accurate or reliable. Misinformation and unverified content circulate widely on the internet, and patients can sometimes feel overwhelmed by conflicting advice, leading to confusion and anxiety. This phenomenon, known as "cyberchondria", can result in patients becoming excessively self-diagnosing or demanding unnecessary treatments, even if they are not endorsed by medical professionals.

Despite these challenges, the overarching trend remains evident: technology has empowered patients to become more knowledgeable and assertive regarding their involvement in healthcare decisions. This presents both a challenge and an opportunity to adapt to an evolving landscape in which patients are no longer passive recipients of care.

I prefer to think that this presents an opportunity for improved healthcare for everyone.

PATIENT-DRIVEN REVOLT AND THE CALL FOR INCLUSION

Once entirely reliant on doctors for information and decision-making, patients are now advocating for greater involvement in their care. This shift away from the traditional, paternalistic healthcare system is driven by several factors, including the desire for transparency, empowerment, and autonomy in managing their health. The increasing demand for inclusion in healthcare decisions is a direct response to a system that has long excluded patients from the decision-making process.

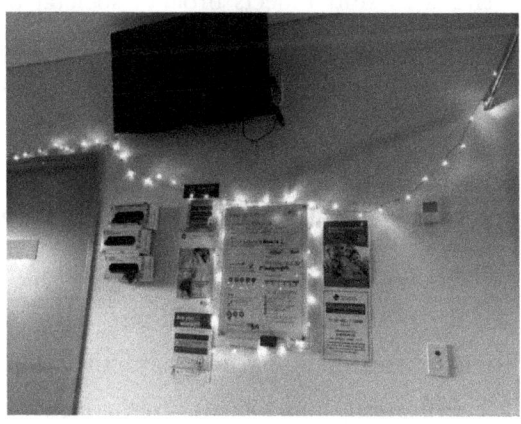

Patient-centred care takes many forms.

Patients wish to feel seen and heard. They seek to have their voices included in the conversation about their treatment and want to believe they are active participants in decisions that affect their bodies and lives.

This feeling of exclusion has been particularly acute in complex medical scenarios where patients grapple with chronic illnesses, rare conditions, or treatments with long-term implications. In these situations, patients seek more than merely a passive receipt of care – they desire collaboration, communication, and respect for their expertise regarding their lives and bodies.

Mikayla's story is precisely that – a complex situation where we anticipated more assistance. When that assistance was lacking, we decided to take matters into our own hands. We became not only active participants but also advocates for uncovering the truth.

THE EXPECTATIONS OF EQUALITY AND AUTONOMY IN HEALTHCARE

The modern patient no longer accepts being relegated to the role of a passive recipient. This shift reflects broader societal trends towards equality, individual rights, and autonomy. Just as movements for inclusivity and participation have transformed other sectors, so too has healthcare.

THE RISE OF THE "EMPOWERED PATIENT"

Empowered patients are informed, engaged, and proactive. They may arrive at a doctor's surgery with a well-researched understanding of their condition or treatment options, and they are ready to ask questions, seek clarification, and discuss alternatives. This newfound autonomy does not reject medical professionals but demands respect and partnership.

THE DEMAND FOR RESPECTFUL, EQUAL RELATIONSHIPS

At its core, the increasing demand for equality in healthcare is a call for respect. Patients desire their humanity to be acknowledged—not merely to be seen as cases to be solved, but as individuals with lives, values, and preferences that must be considered in the treatment process.

Social movements advocating for the rights of marginalised communities have also strengthened this expectation of equal treatment, and patients now anticipate healthcare to embody these values.

In practice, this means healthcare professionals must adjust their approach to ensure that patients are informed and treated as equal partners in their care. Patients are no longer willing to defer entirely to the doctor's judgement. They wish to be involved in the decision-making process, recognising that their lived experiences, personal values, and preferences are crucial to creating a treatment plan that is effective for them.

WHY HEALTHCARE ORGANISATIONS FAIL CUSTOMERS

Despite these evolving expectations, many healthcare organisations let down customers for a variety of reasons. This failure primarily arises from their inability to adapt to the shifting power dynamics between healthcare providers and patients.

Healthcare systems often undergo slow change, primarily due to institutional inertia. Long-established hierarchies, bureaucratic structures, and rigid professional boundaries govern hospital and clinic operations. This leads to a lack of flexibility and responsiveness to patient needs, leaving many patients feeling alienated from their care.

Healthcare organisations often prioritise efficiency, throughput, and cost over patient-centred care. This leads to an impersonal approach to healthcare, where patients are viewed as cases to be resolved rather than individuals with unique needs, expectations, and preferences.

The traditional hierarchical model of authority in healthcare increasingly conflicts with the expectations of modern patients. Many doctors, though well-intentioned, may still project an air of superiority or adopt an authoritarian approach during patient interactions. This can lead to a sense of disempowerment among patients, causing them to feel excluded from decisions that impact their lives. When patients feel dismissed, their trust in the healthcare system wanes.

CULTURAL CHANGE WITHIN HEALTHCARE SYSTEMS

Healthcare organisations must embark on a cultural shift that prioritises patient autonomy and inclusivity. This involves re-evaluating the conventional doctor-patient relationship, breaking down hierarchies, and nurturing an environment of mutual respect and collaboration.

INTEGRATION OF TECHNOLOGY

Leveraging technology will continue to improve communication, streamline processes, and make healthcare more accessible. This includes using patient portals, telemedicine, and AI-driven tools to enhance patient education and care delivery.

The growing demand for equality, autonomy, and inclusion in healthcare indicates a significant shift in the doctor-patient relationship. As patients become increasingly informed, empowered, and engaged in their care, healthcare organisations must adapt to meet these new expectations. Those who fail to acknowledge and respond to this change risk alienating their customers and undermining the trust essential for effective care.

The future of healthcare rests on collaboration, respect, and the recognition that patients are not merely recipients of care but active participants in their own health and well-being. By embracing these values, healthcare systems can keep up with society and enhance their practices.

CHAPTER 34

HOW CAN WE USE TECHNOLOGY TO HELP THE MEDICAL PROFESSION?

The healthcare system is vast and complex, often characterised by fragmented workflows and outdated practices that hinder patient care. Technology is pivotal in addressing the systemic issues in healthcare which have emerged from disjointed information flow, inefficiency, inadequate access to care, and a lack of seamless communication across specialties and departments.

It has the potential to tackle many of these challenges, assisting medical professionals and organisations in enhancing patient care, reducing administrative burdens, and optimising resource use.

Patient data fragmentation is a fundamental issue in healthcare. When information is scattered across various providers, hospitals, or regions, it often results in errors, duplicative testing, delayed diagnoses, and misdiagnoses. This is a complex ICT problem. Maybe the newcomer to ICT can help address this technological issue.

The newcomer is Artificial Intelligence (AI), which can be used in diagnosis and potentially address many of the current challenges.

Technology in diagnosis will be one of the most significant changes in healthcare resulting from technological advances. This is how I refined my "working theory" months before the doctors did. Initially my working theory was the relationship between energy use and seizures. When I used AI this refined the results.

It explains how I managed to stop Mikayla from seizing. There is a glimmer of hope for anyone with undiagnosed conditions. Let's be frank: humans have yet to help successfully.

The use of AI in diagnosis will revolutionise the diagnostic process.

Historically, healthcare has been divided into numerous specialties that focus narrowly on specific aspects of the human body. While this specialisation has undoubtedly led to advancements in medical knowledge, it has also fostered a "not my organ" mentality. Doctors often hesitate to address issues outside their expertise, which can leave patients feeling overlooked or misunderstood.

Multidisciplinary digital platforms can unite specialists from diverse fields to collaboratively treat patients with complex conditions. Virtual meetings, data sharing, and cooperative documentation can dismantle the barriers between specialties, enabling providers to work together on comprehensive care plans that encompass all facets of a patient's health.

AI-enhanced cross-disciplinary diagnosis: This is an exciting use of AI. AI can help doctors bridge gaps between specialties by analysing patient data across multiple domains. For instance, a patient with heart disease may also exhibit neurological symptoms. AI-powered tools can analyse both sets of data concurrently, flagging potential connections and aiding doctors in making more comprehensive, integrated diagnoses.

Teleconsultation for multi-specialty collaboration: Teleconsultation platforms allow specialists from different fields to discuss complex cases without geographical barriers. These collaborative virtual consultations enable a team of specialists to evaluate treatment options, ensuring that every aspect of the patient's condition is addressed.

AI-assisted clinical tasks: Automation and AI can also alleviate healthcare professionals' workloads by automating repetitive tasks, enabling them to concentrate on the more significant aspects of patient care. By incorporating AI into diagnostic imaging, charting, and administrative duties, healthcare professionals can devote more time to patient interaction, thereby enhancing job satisfaction and improving patient outcomes.

Another notable cultural barrier is the resistance to change within the medical field. Many healthcare professionals, particularly those who have been practising for years, may be reluctant to adopt new technologies due to their unfamiliarity, concerns about the reliability of technology, or fears of disrupting established workflows.

Technology holds transformative potential in addressing systemic and cultural barriers within the healthcare system. To fully realise these benefits, the medical profession must adopt a shift in mindset and practice, transitioning from hierarchical, isolated structures to a more integrated, patient-centred approach.

Through a combination of technology, education, leadership, and patient engagement, the healthcare system can evolve into a more efficient, compassionate, and innovative field—one where patients and providers are genuine partners in care. By overcoming resistance and cultural inertia, we can pave the way for a future harmonised with technology and human expertise.

CHAPTER 35

HOSPITAL STRUCTURES AND MIKAYLA'S MEDICAL MISDIAGNOSIS

The behaviour within the hospital could be described as Machiavellian, which reflects their own need to retain power. The consequences to us were tangible and severe.

Leadership and governance in hospitals are crucial components that shape the organisation's strategy, culture, and daily operations. In healthcare, leaders are responsible for ensuring smooth operations and fostering an environment where medical professionals can work collaboratively and efficiently to deliver optimal care.

In a hospital's complex environment, inter-organisational alignment is essential to ensure that various departments and healthcare providers work together effectively to offer coordinated, patient-centred care. However, medical misdiagnoses remain a significant issue even with the best organisational strategies in place.

From my experience as a carer for Mikayla, as a patient myself, and as a professional, I have had the opportunity to see firsthand how and why misdiagnosis occurred for Mikayla. We have also experienced how rigid hierarchies, and institutional biases can hinder further investigation, even when symptoms worsen.

Mikayla was not merely misdiagnosed; medical professionals overlooked her worsening seizures instead of thoroughly investigating them. Each visit to the emergency room followed a predictable pattern: dismissal, insufficient testing, and a reluctance to reconsider the initial diagnosis. The healthcare system's reliance on protocols and hierarchies meant that once a specialist had established a diagnosis, others were hesitant to challenge it, even considering escalating symptoms.

Was being 22 hours unconscious in the ICU not a clear enough warning that something was seriously wrong?

The consequences of stagnant diagnoses

The following happened during Mikayla's 21 emergency department presentations and hospital admissions. The clear evidence came from the patient's mother, but this was even ignored.

- Patients like Mikayla fall into a medical grey area where their condition is deemed "solved" even when clear evidence suggests otherwise.
- Doctors, constrained by hierarchical structures, are reluctant to challenge previous diagnoses out of concern for undermining their colleagues or stepping outside their area of expertise.
- Missed critical opportunities for early intervention resulted in prolonged suffering, unnecessary hospital visits, and heightened healthcare costs.

KAREN PERKS

The need for continuous review and collaboration

- Hospitals should establish interdisciplinary review panels for ongoing and deteriorating conditions.
- A formal escalation pathway should be in place, enabling caregivers to seek a review of prior diagnoses when symptoms persist in deteriorating.
- Patient advocates ought to be empowered to enhance communication between departments and advocate for investigations when necessary.

It is deeply concerning that, even as Mikayla's seizures increased in frequency and severity, the medical system remained inflexible in its initial conclusion. Hospitals should not operate as static institutions where diagnoses are made once and never revisited. Instead, they must adopt a dynamic, patient-centred approach to prevent further instances of prolonged misdiagnosis and medical negligence. What is more worrying is that, if I could figure it out, why couldn't the hospital team?

Mikayla's worsening condition should have prompted a thorough reassessment; however, the rigid adherence to initial – and incorrect – diagnoses overrode clinical judgment. I doubt this is an isolated case but somewhat indicative of a broader culture within healthcare institutions where hierarchies and entrenched beliefs obstruct genuine interdisciplinary collaboration. I made it quite clear that the FND diagnosis was incorrect – telling every doctor, whether they cared to listen or not, and none ever asked why I believed that. The instruction to write "Mother disagrees with diagnosis" in her patient notes indicated a problem. What is wrong, people?

Despite the presence of various specialists and departments, there was a glaring absence of genuine consultation between teams. The lack of a holistic, patient-focused approach resulted in missed crucial opportunities to rectify the diagnosis, leading to further suffering. There was a moment when two specialties argued over whose funding was responsible for the admission.

The consequences of this systemic failure extend far beyond Mikayla's case. People are dying, living in pain, unable to work, and facing financial devastation – all due to a reluctance to challenge authority within the medical hierarchy. Too often, hospital structures prioritise maintaining established power dynamics over fostering a culture of open inquiry and continuous learning. The unwillingness to reassess initial diagnoses arises from a deeply ingrained resistance to questioning senior decision-makers, even when patient outcomes clearly indicate the need for further examination.

It is even more profound than an unwillingness to question. One emergency doctor explained that the system requires them to only refer seizure patients to neurologists—but what happens when neurologists become the problem? There was no ability to request intervention to investigate differently, and calling the REACH line was useless.

Furthermore, the failure to investigate deteriorating conditions serves as a stark reminder of how patient advocacy is frequently overlooked within hospital environments. Families and carers who advocate for additional tests and second opinions often find themselves dismissed or labelled as difficult. This dismissive attitude not only prolongs suffering but also undermines trust in the healthcare system. Hospitals must recognise that patients and their carers are invaluable partners in healthcare and should be actively included in the diagnostic process rather than being marginalised.

Being involved does not mean just communicating a message. It means participating in conversations as the team and making decisions.

It wasn't only Mikayla labelled – she with FND. I too was labelled, as "difficult", and dismissed.

This issue highlights a fundamental misalignment in hospital inter-organisational coordination. Despite hospitals having policies that promote interdisciplinary teamwork, these policies frequently falter in practice due to hierarchical barriers, ineffective communication, and a lack of accountability. Without authentic collaboration between departments and a commitment to prioritising patient outcomes over ego or protocol, misdiagnoses may persist, leading to devastating consequences.

As a mother, and on behalf of all parents and carers, I refuse to accept this status quo. Systemic change is needed to ensure that all voices—especially those of patients and their carers—are heard and valued in medical decision-making. Inter-organisational alignment must move beyond theoretical frameworks and be actively implemented in ways that hold medical professionals accountable for investigating worsening conditions rather than dismissing them.

The fight against medical misdiagnosis is not merely about improving processes; it is about saving lives. We must ask ourselves: How many more Mikaylas must suffer before we dismantle the barriers hindering proper medical investigation? It is time for a cultural shift within healthcare, one that prioritises patient-centred care over rigid hierarchies and ensures that misdiagnoses are not only acknowledged but actively prevented through a commitment to continuous learning and collaborative decision-making.

To achieve genuine change, healthcare institutions must adopt a patient-first mindset, ensuring that processes for reassessment are standardised and mandated when symptoms worsen. Routine interdisciplinary case reviews, enhanced feedback mechanisms, and a willingness to seek second opinions should be integrated into hospital protocols, specifically an independent second opinion, not one from the same hospital. Healthcare workers must be encouraged and empowered to raise concerns when they identify potential misdiagnoses, rather than being pressured to conform to the status quo.

Ultimately, responsibility lies not only with medical professionals but also with policymakers, hospital administrators, and society. A fundamental restructuring of healthcare dynamics is necessary to move away from a system that values authority over accuracy. Until then, patients like Mikayla and their families will continue to bear the consequences of a system that prioritises internal politics over the well-being of those it is meant to serve.

CHAPTER 36

WHAT NEEDS TO CHANGE FIRST TO ADDRESS MEDICAL MISDIAGNOSIS

After spending over 2,000 hours in hospitals, we observed a lot: emergency, neurology, cardiology, ICU, and the other areas of the hospital. My constant thoughts were, "Why am I here?" "What am I supposed to be learning?" I know that things happen for a reason. I wasn't expecting these events and wasn't even considering the why. But here they were, and so for me, I had to absorb, assess, acknowledge, and act.

Our experience revealed several insights, such as the emergency department's excellent performance in trauma cases. It operates as a high-functioning team, with relevant roles and responsibilities working together seamlessly like cogs in a machine. In these circumstances, one can observe how the hierarchical structure functions effectively and successfully.

However, high-performing teams operate within a hierarchy structure. For example, a football team requires a captain to thrive, every athlete relies on a coach, and every business needs a CEO.

But systemic problems arise when power in these roles removes a client- or patient-centred approach to delivery.

There were seven areas that could have significantly positively impacted Mikayla and other cases of misdiagnosis:

1. Integrated technology,
2. Improved communication, and
3. Patient-centred healthcare
4. Patient advocates who can walk in both worlds
5. A three-time emergency department trigger
6. Ensure timely access to your patient records
7. Transparent escalation process for complex medical conditions.

Technology is the fastest way to make a difference. Improved communication and patient experience represent a longer-term strategy. Change is involved—shifting human beliefs and behaviour. But technology—wow—can influence results so much more rapidly.

The complexity of healthcare clearly demonstrated that it requires a multifaceted approach to addressing one of the numerous intricate issues within the sector. Nevertheless, all seven areas for improvement can be classified into one of three categories –

1. Improved technology.
2. Policy and procedures changes.
3. Improved communication across disciplines and teams.

However, nothing on this list is unattainable or out of reach. We merely need to desire the changes we wish to make.

Access to patient records without delays or interference

Current issue: Numerous patients encounter delays in accessing their medical records, which can impede their ability to make informed decisions regarding their care. This frequently results in fragmented care, confusion, or missed opportunities for early intervention.

Secure patient portals empower patients with easy access to their medical records. By giving patients full access to their data, hospitals can increase transparency and trust and enable patients to be more proactive in their care.

Cultivate a culture of transparency, where patients are encouraged to engage with their health information, ask questions, and advocate for their wellbeing.

Benefits

1. Quicker identification of errors or overlooked diagnoses by patients and their family members.
2. Patient satisfaction increases as they feel more involved in the decision-making process.
3. Enhanced management of overall care by empowering patients to monitor their own health data.

Increased use of AI in diagnostics

The fear of relying on AI and other technologies in the diagnostic process can hinder progress in the medical field. Many healthcare professionals may resist these innovations due to concerns about misinterpretation or job displacement. However, AI in medicine is intended to support doctors, not replace them.

AI is not merely a note-taking tool; it harnesses the power to create a far greater impact in achieving health outcomes for many. We must not allow our own fears to obstruct the benefits, particularly when security risks are mitigated.

Enhance the application of AI in diagnostics, particularly in fields like radiology, pathology, and cardiology. AI systems can assist in recognising patterns and proposing potential diagnoses based on extensive datasets, aiding healthcare professionals in making more precise decisions.

Invest in training healthcare professionals to effectively collaborate with AI tools, emphasising that AI is a complementary aid rather than a replacement. Training programmes should highlight AI's capacity to assist in identifying patterns that human eyes alone may overlook.

Ensure that AI systems are consistently updated and assessed for accuracy by utilising diverse and comprehensive datasets to prevent biases.

Benefits

1. Enhanced diagnostic accuracy, especially in intricate or uncommon conditions.
2. Reduced physician burnout as AI assumes routine tasks, enabling healthcare providers to concentrate on critical decision-making.
3. Foster enhanced collaboration between healthcare professionals and AI tools, promoting a culture of innovation rather than fear.

Establishing patient advocates as a systemic resource

Many patients, particularly those with complex or chronic conditions, surely feel unsupported like us or struggle to navigate the healthcare system effectively. This absence of support can result in missed diagnoses, inadequate care coordination, and frustration.

Implement a structured patient advocacy system within hospitals, where trained advocates liaise between patients and medical professionals. Advocates can help patients understand their treatment options, ensure they receive the correct information, and facilitate better communication between patients and healthcare teams.

Establish clear roles for patient advocates within hospital settings, ensuring their involvement in high-risk cases and enabling them to serve as the patient's representative in medical discussions.

Benefits

1. Enhanced communication between patients and healthcare providers, resulting in better-informed decision-making.
2. Decrease stress and confusion for patients, as they have someone to navigate the complex healthcare system with them.
3. Improved patient satisfaction and confidence in the healthcare system.

Three-time emergency department initiate a case-management approach.

Patients who visit the emergency department (ED) numerous times for similar or unresolved issues often slip through the cracks. Without appropriate case management, these patients may remain misdiagnosed or untreated.

After a patient presents to the ED for the same issue multiple times within a defined period (eg number of days), they should be assigned to a case manager, or, if they initiate it, they should need care.

This case manager would review the patient's medical history, organise further investigations, and ensure appropriate specialists are consulted without being tied to a specific specialty. The manager would examine the patient's condition from multiple angles.

Benefits

4. Ensures more thorough care for patients with chronic or complex conditions.
5. Stops patients from being "bounced" between specialists without a precise diagnosis.
6. Lessens the chances of misdiagnosis through a more systematic and coordinated approach to care.

Straightforward escalation process for complex internal medicine cases in public hospitals

Public hospitals frequently experience high patient volumes, resulting in delays in diagnosing and treating intricate internal medicine cases. In these settings, physicians may become inundated with routine cases and overlook the warning signs of more complex conditions.

Establish an escalation process for cases involving complex internal medicine issues. This process should ensure that a senior physician or specialist reviews the patient's case when a diagnosis is unclear or complex.

Establish a protocol for internal referrals that ensures patients receive prompt, multi-disciplinary assessments of their conditions. This process must guarantee that cases with uncertain diagnoses are swiftly escalated for further investigation, rather than being dismissed or left unresolved.

Benefits

1. Ensures that complex cases receive the attention they require, thereby minimising the risk of diagnostic errors.

2. Encourages collaboration between general practitioners and specialists, resulting in more precise diagnoses.
3. Enhances patient outcomes by ensuring that serious conditions are not neglected.

Straightforward escalation process for complex internal medicine cases in the private sector

There are many occasions when misdiagnosis or complex care is not an emergency, but these patients still need advanced care or if left untreated becomes an emergency.

Our experience revealed significant gaps in the system, flaws that allowed misdiagnosis to persist and delayed critical intervention. The lack of interdisciplinary communication was astonishing. Specialists operated in silos; their reports appeared to be lost in a bureaucratic void. Essential information that could have made all the difference was not shared effectively.

This fragmented approach not only delayed treatment but also fostered a sense of disconnect, a feeling that our concerns were falling on deaf ears, that we were merely a statistic, just another case to be checked off a list.

We need greater awareness of the potential for misdiagnosis, not just as a possibility but as a significant risk that requires vigilance and a thorough, multifaceted approach. We must move beyond a symptom-based diagnosis approach and embrace a more holistic, patient-centred perspective. Consider incorporating family observations and patient-reported outcomes into the diagnostic process. Our persistent reports of unusual and changing symptoms were dismissed as irrelevant. We need systems that value and actively solicit this critical information.

Furthermore, the system must provide improved support for families dealing with intricate medical challenges. The emotional toll is immense, and the financial burden is staggering. We have spent countless hours in waiting rooms, accumulating escalating medical bills.

This is not merely a matter of compassion; it is an essential aspect of effective patient care.

The issue of gaslighting – the insidious practice of dismissing or minimising legitimate concerns – must be addressed directly. Medical professionals possess immense power, and that power must be wielded responsibly. A structured process is needed for families to escalate concerns, ensuring their voices are heard and taken seriously, without facing condescending dismissal or outright rejection. Making a complaint to the relevant authority is not the solution.

We require mechanisms to address complaints objectively, investigate allegations of misdiagnosis thoroughly, and hold medical professionals accountable for their actions. This accountability is not about punishment; it is about learning and improving the system to prevent future errors.

Finally, patient empowerment is key. As patients and families, we need to be equipped with the knowledge and resources to advocate for ourselves effectively. This requires accessible educational materials, clear explanations of medical procedures, and support groups where families can share experiences and learn from each other. Informed patients are empowered patients. They are better equipped to ask the right questions, challenge assumptions, and seek second opinions. They are less likely to be swayed by authority and less likely to be silenced by gaslighting.

Our journey has been excruciatingly painful, attesting to the profound impact of medical error. Yet, a determined voice emerges—our voice advocating for improved communication, advanced diagnostic tools, robust support systems, accountability, and patient empowerment. This voice demands systemic change, prioritising the human cost and recognising the profound impact of medical misdiagnosis on individuals, families, and society.

Many may argue that this education is in place. It is not known when you are a patient. Patients and families arriving at ED are not looking to read brochures – for us we were struggling to work out where to go for the first few attendances.

Moreover, the system must recognise and address biases influencing diagnostic decisions. Implicit biases may lead to disparities in care, with specific populations and genders being more likely to receive incorrect or delayed diagnoses. A commitment to diversity and inclusion in the medical profession is essential, ensuring that healthcare providers are adequately trained to recognise and mitigate their biases. This necessitates ongoing education and training, emphasising cultural competence and promoting awareness of health disparities.

The necessity for transparent, easily accessible, and comprehensible medical records is crucial. Our experience revealed the lack of transparency within the medical system, the challenges in accessing and understanding our daughter's medical records, and the frustration of attempting to navigate a complex bureaucratic maze. Patients and their families ought to have immediate and effortless access to their full medical records. This enhanced transparency not only empowers patients but also facilitates better communication and diagnostic accuracy.

Finally, patient advocacy is crucial in ensuring that patients receive timely and accurate diagnoses. Our journey highlighted the importance of patient advocacy, both for our family and for others facing similar situations. There was none in the hospital—it was a management position.

The path ahead is not merely about repairing individual components; it is about fundamentally reshaping the healthcare system. It centres on constructing a system that values collaboration, transparency, and patient-centred care. It seeks to foster a culture of accountability, where errors are addressed openly, learned from, and prevented. It aims to empower patients and families to become active participants in their healthcare, confident in their capacity to advocate for their needs.

Our journey was a nightmare, but we have emerged into a better future from that nightmare. Driving a future in which families no longer must endure the agony of medical misdiagnosis, a future where every patient receives the care they deserve, a future where the human cost of medical error is minimised, and families are heard and genuinely understood and supported.

PART EIGHT

CHAPTER 37

LESSONS LEARNT FROM THE JOURNEY

The initial shock of the misdiagnosis, the relentless cycle of seizures, and the constant fear were the defining features of our early experience. But as the months passed, a strange transformation began to take place. The acute agony gave way to something else, something more challenging to define yet equally powerful: a growing understanding, a deepening empathy, and an unexpected sense of purpose.

We entered this ordeal clinging to hope, but the crucible of our suffering had forged that hope. It wasn't naive, blind optimism but a hard-won conviction that some light could still exist even in the dark corners of despair. This hope was based not on the promises of medical professionals but on our fierce determination to fight for Mikayla. It was a hope nourished by our unshakeable family bonds and the unwavering love we shared.

Our family did not break. We wobbled a couple of times, but we held together and continued today.

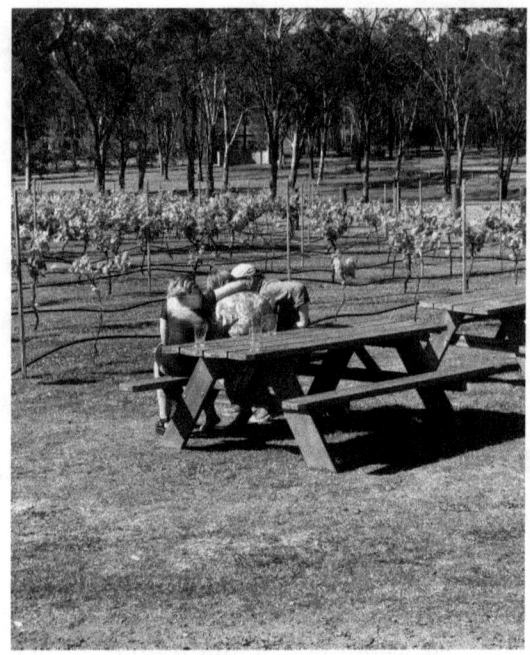

The bond is stronger than ever.

The medical system tested us to our limits with its labyrinthine procedures and often indifferent professionals. Yet, paradoxically, navigating this system became another lesson in resilience. We learnt to advocate fiercely. It wasn't easy to challenge doctors. It goes against my instinct—as I am sure it does many. I trust their knowledge, but knowing what I know now, where does that trust come from? But we all give them the power willingly and without question.

However, in times of trauma and urgent need, we require them – desire them – to wield all this power.

It is confusing our own beliefs regarding this profession.

We uncovered the strength of persistence and the significance of diligent documentation for every interaction, each test result, and every missed opportunity. We transformed ourselves, educated ourselves through medical journals, and became patient advocates armed with the knowledge and resolve to challenge the status quo.

This journey taught me the importance of self-advocacy for myself and others who might find themselves in similar predicaments. Self-advocacy involves learning to listen to your intuition and trust your gut feeling when something doesn't feel right. It also consists of demanding answers, questioning procedures, and refusing to accept dismissive responses from medical professionals. Finally, it involves understanding your rights as a patient and knowing how to use them to get the care you need.

The experience compelled us to confront our vulnerabilities and limitations. We endured moments of profound despair when the weight of our circumstances felt unbearable. There were times we questioned everything, as doubt gnawed at our resolve. Yet, these moments of darkness were not in vain. They acted as a catalyst for growth, revealing the depths of our resilience and the unyielding strength of the human spirit.

Our journey also deepened our understanding of the complexities of medical practice. We learnt that doctors, while undeniably skilled, are not infallible. They are human, and humans make mistakes. While regrettable, these mistakes are not always intentional, reinforcing the importance of patients advocating for themselves. Be strong, be firm, and escalate. The medical system is fraught with imperfections, with protocols and procedures that sometimes prioritise efficiency over patient care.

We encountered compassion and indifference from medical professionals, highlighting the disparities in the quality of care. This experience underscored the crucial need for better communication between doctors and patients and for a system that prioritises transparency and accountability.

Be confident to speak up – you can, as difficult as it may seem.

One of the most profound lessons we learned was the importance of forgiveness. Forgiving ourselves for our shortcomings, for the times when we felt overwhelmed, and for the moments we doubted our abilities to navigate this system was crucial for our healing. Forgiving the medical professionals who had made mistakes—not for their sake, but for ours—was a liberating act. Holding onto anger and resentment only served to prolong our suffering.

Forgiveness was not about condoning their actions; it was about liberating ourselves from the weight of negative emotions that hinder our progress.

The journey profoundly impacted our family dynamic. Our shared adversity forged an unbreakable bond, strengthened by our collective experience. We learnt to lean on one another and support each other in times of crisis. This experience profoundly demonstrated the power of family unity, the enduring strength of love, and the importance of mutual support in facing adversity.

These shared experiences transcended the medical context and strengthened our family's bonds in ways we could never have anticipated. Our family unit remained resilient and unified throughout the ordeal. We communicated openly, shared anxieties, and celebrated small victories, all in the protection of the intervention lounge. This collective spirit helped sustain us throughout the long and arduous process.

Furthermore, this journey stands as a testament to the remarkable resilience of the human spirit. My daughter, despite confronting an almost insurmountable challenge, not only survived but is now on the path to recovery. She can see the trajectory of her life.

Witnessing her strength and spirit has served as a constant source of inspiration and hope for us. It has reaffirmed the power of human resilience in the face of adversity, instilling a powerful sense of perseverance within our family and enabling us to overcome significant obstacles.

Looking back, I see our journey not merely as a string of unfortunate events but as a transformative experience. Our suffering was profound, but it was not without purpose. It instilled in us a deep empathy for others, a commitment to patient advocacy, and a resolve to make a difference in the lives of others who may face similar challenges.

Our experience has fuelled my desire to help others avoid the pitfalls we encountered. This journey is about more than just survival. It's about understanding the intricate workings of the medical system and your rights as a patient. It's about empowerment, finding your voice, and refusing to be silenced.

I want others to know they are not alone. This is a call to action for patients everywhere to stand up, speak out, and fight for the care they deserve. This journey, however challenging, has given me a sense of purpose and a mission to ensure that other families do not have to endure what we did.

The lessons learned resonate far beyond the confines of our personal story. They reflect the importance of diligent research, assertive communication, and unwavering advocacy for one's own health. They highlight the vital role of family support and the healing power of shared experiences. Ultimately, they embody hope, resilience, and the transformative ability to find meaning even in the deepest suffering. The scars remain, serving as reminders of the battles fought and won, a testament to the strength we unearthed within ourselves and the unbreakable bonds of our family. The pain persists, yet it is tempered by the knowledge that we emerged stronger, more compassionate, and more determined to make a difference.

Our story is one of resilience and hope for others navigating the treacherous waters of medical misdiagnosis, serving as a testament to the enduring power of the human spirit.

CHAPTER 38

INSPIRING OTHERS TO SPEAK UP

The number of people misdiagnosed, unable to be diagnosed, harmed, or who have died due to medical misdiagnosis is a national disgrace. How can we be causing more harm to individuals now—despite advancements in technology, skills, and information sharing that ought to elevate the profession—when instead, we have fostered a profession that remains fixated on hierarchy and applauds it?

We speak out to make a difference for the next person. One of my favourite authors, Brené Brown, once stated: "One day you will tell your story of how you overcame what you went through, and it will be someone else's guide for someone else."

Sharing your story is not "dobbing" on the protected profession; it is just a "profession." I deliberately addressed each doctor by their first name to gain some level of balancing the power in the doctor-family relationship. This strategy aimed to convey my expectation of equality. I'm unsure it worked, but I refused to facilitate a significant power imbalance.

A profound and often heartbreaking aspect of misdiagnosis, particularly with complex conditions like functional neurological disorder

(FND), is the emotional isolation it can create for patients. Mikayla frequently felt as though she was contending not only with the physical manifestations of her condition but also with a medical system that failed to recognise or adequately address her symptoms.

In recent years, social media platforms such as TikTok, Instagram, and YouTube have provided a much-needed lifeline for patients who feel isolated due to any illness. The ability to connect with others undergoing similar experiences has created virtual communities where individuals can share their stories, offer support, and provide information on navigating the challenges of living with misdiagnosed or complex health conditions.

The same applies to misdiagnosed patients. Mikayla and Alana discovered numerous TikTok, Instagram, and YouTube stories about doctors misdiagnosing FND. These patients were visually furious – very furious. They comprehend not only the physical symptoms but also the emotional toll that accompanies being misdiagnosed. Social media aids in breaking the silence, nurturing a sense of solidarity and community that would otherwise be lacking.

One of the most powerful aspects of sharing personal experiences is the ability to inspire others to speak out and share their own stories. When patients see others openly discussing their struggles, they feel empowered to do likewise. This growing sense of community helps break down the stigma surrounding complex and misunderstood medical conditions. It challenges the notion that these conditions are merely "all in your head" or that patients exaggerate their symptoms.

When individuals speak out about their health struggles, it not only empowers them to take charge of their health journey but also challenges the healthcare system to listen more attentively. It cultivates an environment where patients are encouraged to share their experiences, seek second opinions, and advocate for themselves.

For many, speaking out is an act of defiance against a system that may have let them down. It also serves to humanise the patient experience, shifting the narrative from patient passivity to active participation in their care.

By sharing personal experiences on social media platforms or in patient support groups, individuals not only validate their own experiences but also foster a ripple effect of empowerment. One person's story can inspire countless others to voice their concerns, share their journeys, and advocate for their health.

Patients can also advocate for changes in the healthcare system by coming together as a community. Collective action can help address systemic issues that contribute to misdiagnosis.

The rise of social media has provided patients who are misdiagnosed or living with complex conditions an opportunity to find support, education, and community in ways that were once unattainable. These platforms have established virtual spaces for individuals to share their experiences, empower others, and advocate for systemic change.

As patients continue to voice their concerns, they not only encourage others to do likewise but also foster a cultural shift towards more open, patient-centred healthcare. By sharing their stories, providing educational resources, and advocating for improved care, individuals transform their struggles into a collective force for change. Through this empowerment and solidarity, patients can overcome the isolation of misdiagnosis and collaborate to create a healthcare system that is more inclusive, transparent, and responsive to their needs.

CHAPTER 39

WHERE TO FROM HERE?

For 18 months, the only anchor I had was the thought: this cannot happen again to another family. The grim and saddening reality is that without change, it will. I often sat in silence beside Mikayla, reflecting on what I could do to leave a legacy from this harrowing experience so that the next family feels a little less stressed, a little more empowered, and receives much better support.

Change is necessary—real, tangible change—not just awareness but systemic shifts that prevent others from enduring the same struggles we faced. There are several ways to create meaningful change, but two key initiatives stand out: law reform and charity to support those requiring medical support—those who fall between the systems.

One crucial law change would be ensuring everyone has noncombative access to their patient records. In our journey, we encountered numerous obstacles, including delays in information transfer from one doctor to another. These delays had consequences: Vital details were lost, patterns were missed, and the opportunity for early diagnosis was squandered.

Had we been able to access Mikayla's complete medical records without restriction, it would have contributed to the information we otherwise needed to gather – enabling another professional to identify what had been overlooked.

Transparency in medical records is not merely a convenience but a necessity. Patients and their families should not have to leap through hoops or encounter resistance when seeking information. An open-access approach would result in fewer gaps, fewer delays and, ultimately, better patient outcomes.

This longer-term strategy will rely on raising funds to support those in need. We will prioritise women, children, regional and remote areas, Aboriginal and Torres Strait Islander people, CALD, LGBTIQA+, veterans, and other priority groups.

The model is for AI technology will work alongside doctors to analyse patient data, identifying potential conditions and providing differential diagnoses. This is the future, and we aim to capitalise on using AI for good through research and analysis.

Beyond immediate patient support, I envision a long-term impact in the form of medical trials for the advancement of technology, analysis, and reform. This experience has been profoundly eye-opening and humbling, and it is essential that the lessons learned do not go to waste. That would be an atrocity, wasting two years of Mikayla's life, Alana's life, and my life.

Book 2 – The Voices of Others

This book compiles stories from other patients and families who have faced similar battles within the healthcare system. Their experiences, struggles, and triumphs shed light on systemic failures and the resilience required to overcome them. It would serve as both validation and advocacy, illustrating that these issues are not isolated but widespread. Even now, there are people ready to tell their stories.

Book 3 – Analysing the System Through Research
This would be a study, a deep dive into the organisational and systemic issues within the medical field. From the bureaucratic red tape to the culture of dismissal that often surrounds complex diagnoses, this book would examine where and why the system fails. It would incorporate expert insights, case studies, and data analysis to depict the areas that demand reform clearly.

Book 4 – The Road to Solutions: Through Research
Identifying and advocating for concrete solutions to the issues uncovered in the previous books. This would include policy recommendations, comparisons of healthcare models from other countries, and innovative approaches to patient advocacy. The aim would be to highlight the problems and actively work towards change.

Each of these books would contribute to the broader mission: ensuring that no family must endure what we experienced. They would serve as both a guide and a rallying cry, inspiring individuals, medical professionals, and policymakers to demand and implement meaningful change.

The driving force behind all these efforts is simple: no one should have to fight this hard to be heard, believed, or receive the care they need. The stress, frustration, and sheer emotional toll of battling the medical system should not be a universal experience.

If this journey has taught me anything, it is that change is necessary and possible. We cannot be mediocre, and we cannot afford to accept the status quo. We must push forward, creating a future where families are supported, diagnoses are timely, and the medical system functions as it should: to heal, help, and provide answers.

This is my legacy. This is what I will fight for.

CHAPTER 40

THE PERSONAL THANK YOU

This book would not have been possible without the unwavering support of numerous individuals. First and foremost, I wish to thank my family—my children, Mikayla, Alana, and Reece—whose strength, resilience, and lasting love carried us through this harrowing ordeal. Their courage inspired this book, and their steadfast belief in me fuelled its completion.

Thank you to my family; it would have been a much longer and more arduous journey without you. I am grateful to my friends, who are always listening and there for me. I would also like to thank my clients—those who didn't judge or question my working from a hospital ward.

I am deeply grateful to our GP, Dr Jacob Duvenage, and specialists: Dr John Malcolm, Dr Sahil Vohra, Dr Kirsten Murray, and Dr Magnus Halland; as well as the doctors and nurses who excelled; the management, doctors, and nursing staff at Newcastle Private Hospital ICU and Coronary Care Unit, whose compassion and understanding provided much-needed reassurance of quality care.

These people are the reason Mikayla is healthy again. Their empathy and willingness to listen, even when faced with overwhelming challenges, are testaments to the medical profession's humanity. Their expertise, commitment to patient rights, and listening to the family were instrumental in helping us navigate the complex healthcare system.

There was one pivotal moment that changed Mikayla's entire trajectory. When Dr Sahil Vohra asked a straightforward question after listening to me explain energy use and the seizures –with my spreadsheet on my lap, of course. 'Has anyone suggested a Continuous Blood Glucose Monitor?' Eight words. That is all it took—one doctor to ask eight simple words. I am sure he doesn't appreciate the magnitude of those words. But that is the power of listening.

My gratitude extends to my editor, Karen Weaver, and the team at KMD Books for their guidance, patience, and belief in this story. I sincerely appreciate their dedication to ensuring this book reaches its intended audience. Their unwavering belief in me and this project made all the difference.

And the heaviest question: would I change anything? Absolutely not. The future can be changed. Come with us.

GLOSSARY

This glossary defines key medical and legal terms used throughout the book. We provide definitions in plain language to ensure accessibility for all readers.

EEG (electroencephalogram): A test that measures electrical activity in the brain.

HCCC: Health Care Complaints Commission

FND: Functional neurologic disorder (FND) refers to a neurological condition caused by changes in how brain networks work, rather than changes in the structure of the brain itself.

Gas lighting: Manipulate (someone) using psychological methods into questioning their own sanity or powers of reasoning.

Informed consent: The process by which a patient gives permission for medical treatment after receiving adequate information about the risks and benefits.

Medical malpractice: Professional negligence by a healthcare provider resulting in harm to a patient.

Misdiagnosis: The incorrect identification of a patient's medical condition.

MRI (magnetic resonance imaging): A medical imaging technique that uses a magnetic field and radio waves to create detailed images of the body.

NUM: Nurse Unit Manager

Patient advocate: An individual or organisation that champions patient rights and helps patients navigate the healthcare system.

Rapid response provider: the clinical team or individual responsible for providing emergency assistance to patients whose condition is deteriorating.

Seizure: A sudden, uncontrolled electrical disturbance in the brain.

TEDx: *TEDx* is a grassroots initiative, created in the spirit of TED›s overall mission to research and discover "ideas worth spreading."

AUTHOR BIOGRAPHY

Karen Perks is an entrepreneur with businesses in Australia and the United Kingdom. She specialises in strategic business tender and grant writing. She is also a published author who has contributed to anthologies such as *Courage and Confidence* and *Hear Us Roar*. The latter will be developed into a ten-book series and a docufilm for Apple TV.

Karen's personal experience with the medical misdiagnosis of her daughter, Mikayla, inspired her to write *Mum, Please Help Me*, a moving memoir advocating for patient rights and better communication within the healthcare system.

Through this work, Karen seeks to empower others facing similar challenges with the confidence and resilience required to navigate the complexities of healthcare. She aims to inspire positive change in medical practices, ultimately fostering improved patient outcomes and a more responsive, compassionate healthcare system.

www.ingramcontent.com/pod-product-compliance
Lightning Source LLC
Chambersburg PA
CBHW051534020426
42333CB00016B/1931